The "T"Zone
Health And Fitness
Sports Energy and Nutrition

Manuel F. Forero, M.D., FACC, FACP

authorHOUSE®

AuthorHouse™
1663 Liberty Drive, Suite 200
Bloomington, IN 47403
www.authorhouse.com
Phone: 1-800-839-8640

First published by AuthorHouse 1/27/2008

ISBN: 978-1-4343-5084-8 (sc)

Printed in the United States of America
Bloomington, Indiana

This book is printed on acid-free paper.

DEDICATION

This book is dedicated to all the people who, day in and day out contribute to a deeper and wholesome understanding of my "True-Self." (Mind, Body, and Spirit). To all of you I owe my love and gratitude.

A portion of the proceeds from this book go to support the Health Care programs of Mama Maria Clinic,Kenya, Africa.

mamamaria.org

ACKNOWLEDGEMENTS

I want to give thanks to my parents, my wife and children for their love, patience, and understanding. To the late Manuel M. Forero, M.D., my dad, my mentor, coach, and professor, with whom I shared the soccer ball as a child and later on in medicine, the classroom and the scalpel.

I would like to acknowledge and express my gratitude to Mrs. Yvonne Guerriero for her gracious and unselfish hours of transcription work that made this manuscript possible, to Mr. John Fleming for his unconditional help in the making of the illustrations and to Mrs. Rachel A. Scofield for her creative talent with the art work on the front cover of this book.

I would like to express my most sincere gratitude to the AuthorHouse team for their hard work and dedication in the creation of this book.

INTRODUCTION

My career as a doctor of medicine has given me tremendous joy and health awareness. Having developed the "T" Zone Health and Fitness Cycling Training Program with you in mind, I realized that a more in depth discussion on sports energy and nutrition was to follow.

For over 27 years I have been talking to patients about healthy lifestyle, diet habits and the benefits of exercise. This book is targeted for those who believe in staying healthy. This book is for you, who have already taken the steps to rediscover your body and your potential. The health benefits of exercise are indisputable as well as the joy that goes along with it, but as we know, it is a very personal experience; as personal as the gentle touch of a sunset, the amazement of a starry night, or the warm feeling in the company of a loved one.

This is not a book to lose weight or a book on diets and cardiovascular disease or epidemiology. There are excellent reviews of these topics in my references list. This book is what you and I need to eat and drink to be able to exercise and stay healthy. This book is not for the professional high elite athlete, nor for people with ailments or specific health issues that may need specialized evaluation, counseling and treatment. I hope to reach you with my message. If you fuel properly you will perform properly and stay healthy.

This book is organized into four main sections. Each section takes you in a step wise approach, starting with a basic understanding of energy, what we are as an "Energy Concept," and the energy metabolic systems that generate the power for physical activity and exercise.

The second section gives an in-depth understanding of the basic nutrients or fuel necessary to run the energy metabolic systems with great emphasis on the high quality and least contaminated sources. This section will give you an understanding of why life without water is not possible. Here, you will learn about dehydration and other clinical situations encountered, not infrequently, in the athletic field such as body temperature de-regulation and ways to prevent or treat them as they occur. You will also take a glimpse at some facts on ergogenic aids and the placebo effect.

Section three is a concise, up-to-date and to the point review of the nutrition/hydration needed for optimal exercise performance. More specifically, you will find yourself planning what you will need to eat and drink prior to or during training and competition. Depending on the duration and the intensity of the event, you will learn when water might be more important than fuel and why some athletic events require plenty of both.

The last section shows you why proper diet and exercise leads to a body in harmony and why body composition and ideal strength-to-weight ratio will translate into optimal athletic performance. Keeping a balanced energy expenditure yields physical well being, ideal body weight and healthier lives.

I am confident that this book, if nothing else, will be an eye opener and will increase your awareness of why some people choose to live healthier and feel good about themselves. You have to have the drive and commitment to stay healthy . . . within us is the power of intention.

Contents

PART A: The Energy Systems

PART B: Nutritional Sources

PART C: Training and Recovery Nutrition/ Hydration

PART D: Body Composition / Energy Balance

Health

&

PART A: The Energy Systems

Fitness

I. THE ENERGY CONCEPT

Is Einstein's $E=mc^2$ related to ATP, the universal currency of energy of life on earth? I think so and let me tell you why I think the way I do.

Throughout life our human body is concerned with energy changes in molecular events. ATP has a usable energy content of about 12 kcal/mol. Therefore, whatever created the "Big Bang" created energy. People and scientists have been talking about subatomic "particles," the quarks, the ghost particles (neutrinos), the force particles (gluons, photons, etc.) and now we are talking "superstring" theory and strings of energy and multiple dimensions. Scientists are pulling their hair in an attempt to understand creation and, in fact, some have even said, "understand the mind of God."

We've been taught about the building blocks, "the atoms," that are both mass and energy. Well, orderly clumped atoms lead to molecules, orderly clumped molecules lead to macromolecules (protein, lipid, carbohydrate), to cells, to tissues, to organs, to organisms, to the human body....... to universal consciousness.

The four known forces of the universe include gravity, electromagnetism, the strong force (which holds protons, neutrons, and nuclei together) and the weak force (which is involved in the formation of the chemical elements). Scientists are working now on the "unified field theory" or theory of everything in an attempt to understand gravity in relation to the other three forces of the universe.

We are the universe! Millions of years ago, the conditions that existed on earth were quite different from those of today. However, there is a general agreement that planet earth was a violent place with little, if any, free oxygen (and no ozone layer), volcanic eruptions, lightening, torrential rains, and continued bombardment of ultraviolet radiation from the sun. A perfect natural "laboratory milieu" where certain mixture of gases such as carbon dioxide (CO_2), methane (CH_4), ammonium (NH_4), and hydrogen (H_2) in the presence of hot water, electrical discharges and ultraviolet radiation reacted to form simple organic molecules. These molecules were constructs of carbon (C), hydrogen (H), and nitrogen (N), which upon further reactions and millions of years, now in the presence of oxygen, gave rise to small organic molecules, unicellular organisms, and subsequently to humans. Some of these molecules are amino acids (protein building blocks), carbohydrates (fuel), lipids (energy storage), and nucleotides (building blocks of the genetic code – DNA and RNA). Self replication was of utmost importance to sustain and maintain life. Phosphorus (P) became a player in the generation of ATP (Adenosine tri-phosphate), which is the "energy currency" of human molecular events. Two proteins, actin and myosin, present in our hearts and muscles are coupled in perfect harmony, which when ATP activated, lead to contraction and relaxation. With exercise they get stronger and smarter. When these proteins are absent or defective in humans, it leads to some forms of cardiomyopathy that can lead to heart failure and death and to some forms of muscular dystrophy, very incapacitating indeed.

So let me ask you a question: Is the isolated neuron (brain cell) smarter than the isolated cardiomyocyte (heart cell) or skeletal muscle (muscle cell) or sperm cell (male reproductive) or the oocyte (female reproductive)? Is the immune cell an outsider or are they "team players" for the good and welfare of the whole? Without one or the other we would perish, unable to procreate, to think, to fight infections and out of control "rebel cells" (cancer cells), to pump blood or to exercise – it would be pandemonium.

So who tells them to be "team players?" Despite their uniqueness, individuality and differences, is there a master mind that knows better and knows it all? Or is it all molecules? What are molecules anyway? Aren't they energy? The wisdom of creation... isn't it?

II. ENERGY METABOLIC SYSTEMS

Working muscles need energy. Energy is neither created nor destroyed, but rather transformed from one form to another according to the first law of thermodynamics. The energy supplied for working muscles is derived from two systems: The aerobic and the anaerobic. The contribution of each system is directly related to exercise intensity and duration. Please refer to figure 1.

Figure 1 ***Aerobic and Anaerobic Systems***

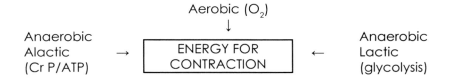

Aerobic (O_2)
↓
Anaerobic Alactic (Cr P/ATP) → **ENERGY FOR CONTRACTION** ← Anaerobic Lactic (glycolysis)

The different metabolic systems may (aerobic) or may not (anaerobic) use oxygen (O_2) and may (lactic) or may not (alactic) accumulate lactate. Where does lactate come from? From the breakdown of glucose in what is known as the glycolytic system of which we will be talking more about as we go along. All energy for muscle contraction is provided both by creatine phosphate (Cr P) and Adenosine tri-phosphate (ATP), the universal currency of energy. One mole (mol) represents the molecular weight of a substance in grams. The concentration ratio of stored Cr P/ATP in the cell ranges from 3:1 to 6:1. Approximately five millimoles (mmol) of ATP and 15 millimoles (mmol) of creatine phosphate are stored within each kilogram of muscle. Very short and maximum intensity workloads (i.e., 100-yard dash) will deplete the storage of Cr P and ATP within 10 seconds, though, once the physical activity is over, Cr P and ATP are replenished within a few minutes. Replenishment is 70% complete within 30 seconds and 100% after 3-5 minutes. The system does not use oxygen (anaerobic) and does not generate lactate (alactic). This system is known as the anaerobic alactic system. See figure 2.

Figure 2 ***Anaerobic Alactic System***

$$\text{ATP} \underset{}{\overset{\text{ATPase}}{\rightleftharpoons}} \text{ADP + P + ENERGY (mechanical work)}$$

$$\text{Cr P} \underset{}{\overset{\text{Cr kinase}}{\rightleftharpoons}} \text{Cr + P + ENERGY (mechanical work)}$$

After a few months of endurance training (i.e., cycling or running three to four times a week) stores of Cr P and ATP increase by 25 to 50%. Eight weeks of sprint training resets the anaerobic alactic system by increasing the enzymes that break down and reconstitute ATP and Cr P, thereby speeding both energy release and ATP regeneration.

In skeletal muscle the Type II (fast-twitch) muscle fibers are predominantly the ones undergoing the structural and biochemical changes just discussed, particularly so, the Type II-B muscle fibers. These cells are mostly anaerobic with a low oxidative capacity. They can perform above the anaerobic threshold (AT) during short and intense bursts of energy (seconds). In a typical sprinter, the ratio of Type II (fast-twitch) to Type I (slow-twitch) muscle fibers is 50/50.

However, with a well structured program, sprinters can develop their endurance capacity by recruiting Type II-A fibers. These fibers can supply aerobic energy in addition to their predominant anaerobic function.

Carbohydrate is almost entirely the only macronutrient whose stored energy can be used to generate ATP anaerobically. This is known as the Glycolytic pathway. The complete breakdown of one molecule of glucose yields 36 moles of ATP. The complete breakdown of one molecule of neutral fat (triglyceride with 3: 18-carbon fatty acid) yields 460 moles of ATP almost entirely aerobically. Hence, more energy is obtained from burning fat in the presence of oxygen. However, the limiting factor is oxygen supply. Thereby, fat is not a very economic fuel.

The aerobic metabolic system is designed to obtain energy (ATP) from the breakdown of carbohydrates, fat, and protein in the presence of oxygen. Millions of years ago, none to very little oxygen was available on planet earth. From the evolutionary standpoint glycolysis represents a more primitive form of energy transfer which was all that was needed back then. This anaerobic system is still well developed in some reptiles, amphibians, fish, and diving mammals. Today we can't survive without oxygen.

So, how do I train my aerobic (oxygen) system? By performing intermediate to prolonged (1 to 6 hours) exercise work loads at moderate to moderately high intensities. When we exercise at this level, we do not accumulate lactate. Energy supply is mostly coming from fat oxidation and to a lesser extent, from carbohydrate breakdown (glycolysis). This predominant fat oxidation is taking place in the slow-twitch (Type I) muscle fibers which, as we know, have a high oxidative capacity. They perform below the anaerobic threshold during prolonged exercise loads. We have such tremendous stored energy in fats that theoretically you could bicycle for more than 1,000 miles without exhausting this reserve.

When the work loads become of shorter duration and high intensity, we are training our anaerobic lactic system and we are building up lactate that leads to rapid underperformance and prompt muscle fatigue. Like the anaerobic alactic system, the anaerobic lactic system is best trained with high intensity work loads lasting 1 to 5 minutes. Depending on the athlete's level of conditioning, recovery periods should be active at relatively lower intensities and they can last from 1 minute to 5 to 7 minutes. Table 1 summarizes the basic energy metabolic systems.

TABLE 1 ENERGY METABOLIC SYSTEMS

ENERGY SYSTEM	FUEL SOURCE	DURATION/INTENSITY
AEROBIC		
A. Aerobic	FAT-glucose-ADP-O_2 ↓ ATP	Prolonged/low moderate (240-600 seconds)
B. Aerobic	glucose-fat-ADP-O_2 ↓ ATP	Intermediate/moderately high (120-240 seconds)
ANAEROBIC		
A. Anaerobic Lactic (Glycolytic)	GLUCOSE-ADP ↓ Lactate - ATP	Short/high (10-120 seconds)
B. Anaerobic Alactic	Cr P – ATP	Very short/maximum (1-10 seconds)

A long distance cyclist or marathon runner has a predominance of Type I (slow-twitch) muscle fibers. In fact, some scientists have calculated the Type I to Type II muscle fiber ratio to be 90/10. What is rather interesting is the fact that endurance athletes cannot change these fiber ratios by performing sprint interval workouts. So basically you have a genetic makeup to either be a sprinter or an endurance athlete. As a sprinter you can train to build up more endurance, but not the other way around. The ratios of Type I (slow-twitch) to Type II (fast-twitch) muscle fibers however, may vary considerably among people and cultures throughout the world.

We are all familiar with the overwhelming worldwide dominant endurance marathon runners from Eastern Africa as opposed to the highly selected group of sprinters from the Western part of Africa. Genetic endowment, indeed!

We are constantly generating lactate. Whether we are sleeping or awake, lactate is always there. We have a perfect balance of lactate production and consumption. At high exercise intensities lactate consumption cannot keep up with lactate production and the balance is lost leading to lactate accumulation. This is known as the lactate threshold point or OBLA (onset of blood lactate accumulation). This lactate threshold (La T) correlates well with different physiologic variables that can be determined in the field or in the exercise laboratory. These physiologic variables include the heart rate (HR), the maximal oxygen consumption per unit time (VO_2 max) and the maximal power output which in cycling and other sports is measured in watts (W). While it is true that all of these physiologic variables correlate very well with your training intensities, most people do not need exact La T, VO_2max, or power output (W) determination to see improvement in their training. Though in the exercise physiology laboratory these parameters are very important and are utilized to effectively plan an exercise program in high-profile athletes.

During the grueling Tour de France, athletes will monitor progress and exercise intensities during the actual three weeks of this phenomenal athletic event with the use of the heart rate monitor. At CTS (Carmichaels' Training Systems) they have developed a CTS field test based on percent of CTS field test average heart rates and, in fact, it turns out it works out very well. According to Chris Carmichael: "this is what most people really need; athletes continue to achieve their goals, from gaining fitness to losing weight, and from finishing their first 10K run to winning the Tour de France."

Maximizing the rate of energy production per unit time, for the length of the event, is at the core of "athletic performance" and this is directly related to the rate of lactate production and consumption. This results from the specific interaction, balancing, and level of training of both the aerobic and anaerobic systems.

Figure 3 shows the physiologic correlate of lactate threshold and power output in three different individuals with different levels of fitness.

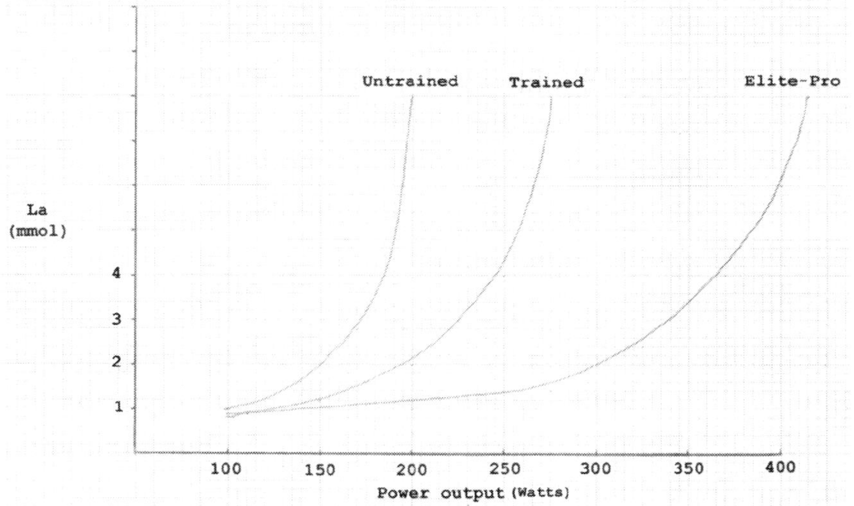

Fig. 3 Physiologic correlate of Lactate threshold (LaT) and Power output (W) in three different individuals with three different levels of fitness.

The athlete to the right can generate more power before the onset of blood lactate accumulation. The untrained individual on the other hand, accumulates lactate earlier, at much lower exercise intensities. The trained individual is somewhere in between.

The physiologic correlate of lactate threshold (LaT), heart rate (HR), power output (W) and energy metabolic systems can be seen in figure 4.

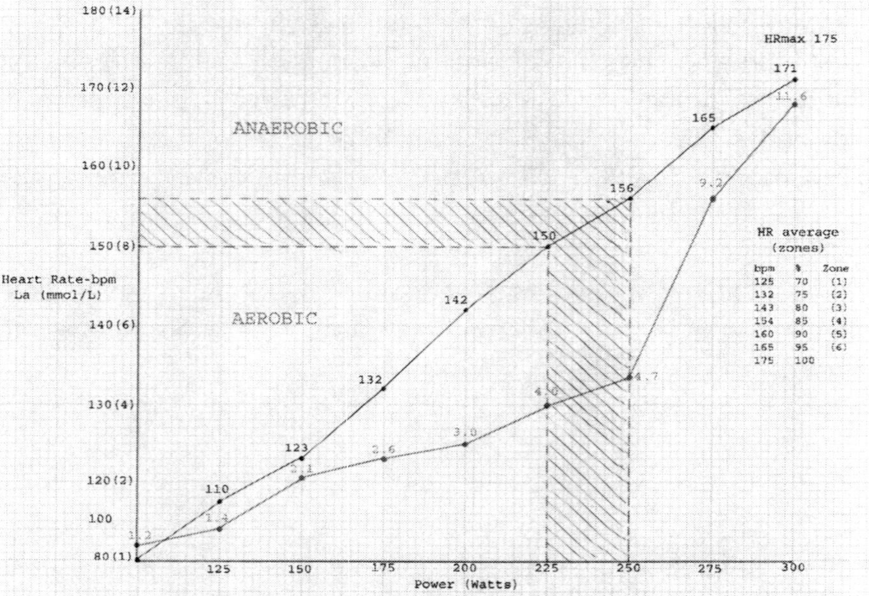

Fig. 4 Physiologic correlates of lactate threshold (LaT), heart rate (HR), power output (W), energy metabolic systems (Aerobic & Anaerobic) and heart rate training zones.

The new international classification of intensity training zones is based on the contributions of the aerobic and anaerobic metabolic systems. The *aerobic zone* energy supply is 100% dependent on oxygen. The *endurance zone* energy supply is part aerobic and part anaerobic. The *anaerobic zone* is almost 100% lactic or alactic (Cr P/ATP).

In my book on exercise performance and physiologic evaluation of the athlete we will do a more in depth review on this subject.

A1 (aerobic 1):	Low to moderate intensity -- at 75 +/- 5% of LaT
A2 (aerobic 2):	Moderate intensity -- at 85 +/- 5% of LaT
E1 (endurance 1)	Moderately high to high intensity -- at 95 +/- 5% of LaT
E2 (endurance 2)	High intensity -- at 100 +/- 5% of LaT
An1 (anaerobic 1)	Short/very high intensity -- 3-5 minutes -- at >100% of LaT
An2 (anaerobic 2)	Very short/maximal intensity -- 10-15 seconds – alactic

III. ENERGY EXPENDITURE

Energy expenditure refers to the amount of energy required to sustain all chemical reactions within the human body. The total daily energy expenditure includes all involuntary bodily functions (basal – resting metabolic rate and energy metabolism of food ingestion) and the energy accounted for by voluntary bodily functions (exercise). This requires a precise and delicate balance of fuel supply (food), water, different vitamins, minerals, micronutrients, and oxygen supply and consumption.

We consume food for two reasons:

1. They provide the essential building blocks of our physical being.
2. They provide the energy necessary to live and perform work.

Food calorie refers to the amount of energy a particular food can deliver to the "power engines" in our cells known as the mitochondria. There is a popular misconception regarding foods "caloric supply." People worry about "fat calories" or "carb calories" thinking that one or the other is good or bad for you or one or the other is going to make you gain or lose some weight. The bottom line is, the more calories we consume the more weight we gain, particularly so if we do not burn them due to lack of exercise. This is a big epidemic in America today. It is estimated that the proportion of North Americans who are moderately overweight has reached a 35-40% staggering figure. What is worse and what has changed dramatically is the overwhelming one-third of Americans which fall within the obesity category (BMI greater than 30). Obesity among children is on the rise, which is an alarming trend and something that needs immediate action. It is estimated that the U.S. spends more than 90 billion dollars a year on medical care for obesity and its complications. I will be talking more about ideal body weight and body mass index at the end of the book.

With meals we consume different amounts and combinations of carbohydrates, lipids, and proteins that will determine our caloric intake; 1 gram of carbohydrate yields 4 kcal, 1 gram of protein yields 4 kcal, and 1 gram of fat yields 9 kcal. Even though the absolute caloric supply per gram of fat is higher than it is for either carbohydrates or protein, carbohydrates more efficiently generate energy per unit of oxygen consumed. In other words, one liter of oxygen yields approximately 5 kcal from the breakdown of 1 gram of carbohydrate, while only 4.7 kcal from the breakdown of 1 gram of fat. Hence, fat is not a very efficient fuel. More oxygen is required in the combustion of 1 gram of fat. The energy expenditure while sleeping, laying down, or sitting while I write this paragraph is minimal, though the vast majority comes from burning fat. Even though the proportion or percentage of fat being burned is high, the absolute volume is very low. As physical activity increases, and particularly so when the exercise intensity is high, the proportion of fat required for energy decreases, while the proportion of energy derived from carbohydrates increases. At high or very high intensity exercise efforts, the total caloric requirement (volume) per unit time is also higher, therefore, the total calorie requirements provided by carbohydrates and fat is higher as well. A small amount of energy is derived from protein breakdown. This book on sports energy and nutrition is focused on this premise. How best to deliver fuel (food, water, and nutrients) to the working muscles and ways to optimize storage and delivery during training, competition, and recovery.

The basal or resting metabolic rate (BMR) is the energy required to maintain all involuntary bodily functions, while at complete rest or during sleep, in a normal otherwise healthy individual. This refers to the energy required to maintain body temperature, neuro endocrine function, respiration, circulation, digestion of food and sustain basal muscle tone. These functions (all involuntary) account for 70% of our daily energy expenditure. The rest (30%) is accounted for by physical activity (voluntary). Working a desk job does not increase your energy expenditure by much. To burn calories you have to move and the more you move, the more you burn. The energy generated by muscle activity can increase nearly 120 times with maximal exercise.

In a normal healthy individual at rest, there is a relatively fixed uptake of oxygen per unit time known as oxygen consumption (VO_2) which is relatively constant at 3.5ml/kg/min. This is also known as one metabolic equivalent (1 MET). The working muscle can increase the oxygen consumption up to 10-15 times and, in professional cyclists, or marathon runners, up to or close to 25 times. This maximum increase in oxygen consumption is also known as VO_2 max which can be measured directly or indirectly in the exercise laboratory.

The main goal of aerobic and endurance training is to increase the amount and intensity of work performed while burning fat and carbohydrates in the presence of oxygen before the onset of blood lactate accumulation. Some athletes experience the shift from aerobic to a predominant anaerobic metabolism, particularly so in the early stages of training, hence, there is early lactate accumulation at low to moderate work intensities (50-70% of VO_2 max). After months or years of training, the same individual might be able to perform high intensity workouts before the onset of blood lactate accumulation at 85 to 90% of maximum effort.

From now on I will concentrate on the fuel characteristics of carbohydrates, lipids (fats), proteins, and the very important participation of vitamins, minerals, micronutrients and water. The human body is an aqueous universe and without water life is not possible. This water represents approximately 70% of a person's total body weight. Sixty-five percent of this water is inside the cells (intracellular) and the remaining 35% is outside the cells (extracellular).

Health

&

PART B: Nutritional Sources

Fitness

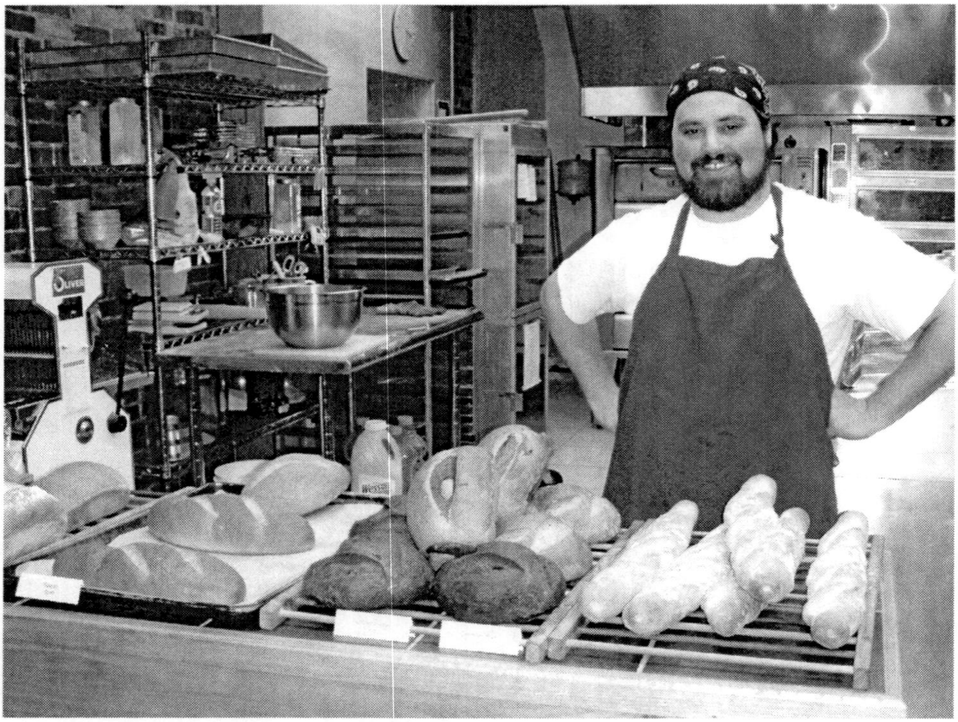

Wheat turned into bread. Smart people know a good source of calories.

I. CARBOHYDRATES

The basic structural unit of carbohydrates is a six carbon molecule with oxygen and hydrogen atoms attached to it. This molecule is a single molecule unit known as monosaccharide. Glucose is a monosaccharide, and the single most important fuel for our bodies. There are two additional monosaccharides known as fructose and galactose. It is the number of monosaccharides bonded together that allows us to classify carbohydrates into simple and complex carbohydrates. For the athlete, carbohydrates are the back bone of their nutritional program. There is no such thing as a bad carbohydrate for the athlete. However, depending on the type of carbohydrate consumption, you can also increase the nutritional value or obtain energy very quickly, whereas others will give you long lasting and slow energy release for the working muscles. Glucose is the fuel that runs both down the anaerobic and aerobic energy metabolic systems and is stored in the liver and skeletal muscle as glycogen. The brain is so dependent on the continuous influx of glucose that no insulin is required to transfer glucose into the brain cells. The monosaccharides are single-molecule units obtained from the breakdown of the disaccharides, which are essentially two connected monosaccharides. There are three main disaccharides – sucrose, lactose, and maltose. Sucrose, also known as cane sugar, contains glucose and fructose as monosaccharides. Lactose, also known as milk sugar, contains glucose and galactose as monosaccharides. Maltose, also known as malt sugar, contains two glucose molecules. The monosaccharides (single-molecule carbohydrates) and the disaccharides (two-molecule carbohydrates) are referred to as simple carbohydrates, or simply sugars. Three or more (20+) molecule carbohydrates are referred to as complex carbohydrates. The complex carbohydrates are digestible, partially digestible or indigestible. This last group is also commonly known as dietary fiber. Please see tables 2 and 3. Finally there are nutritive sweeteners known as sugar alcohols (mannitol, sorbitol, and xylitol).

All carbohydrates, with the exception of the indigestible, nonabsorbable polysaccharides, are broken down to the basic metabolic (fuel) unit for human cells, glucose.

Glucose is stored in the liver and skeletal muscle as glycogen. Glycogen is readily available to maintain blood glucose levels within the relatively narrow range of 70 to 110mg/dl. This is true only for liver glycogen. Muscle glycogen is readily available to the working muscle and will be used both via the aerobic and anaerobic pathways. Even when muscle glycogen stores are full, if the liver glycogen is depleted, the blood glucose levels are not easily maintained.

TABLE 2 SIMPLE CARBOHYDRATES (SUGARS)

MONOSACCCHARIDES	DISACCHARIDES
Glucose (known as dextrose)	Maltose (glucose + glucose)
Fructose (fruit sugar)	Sucrose (fructose + glucose)
Galactose	Lactose (galactose + glucose)

Glucose molecules are rapidly absorbed into the blood stream raising blood sugar and insulin faster and higher. All sugars are easily digested carbohydrates.

TABLE 3 COMPLEX CARBOHYDRATES (POLYSACCHARIDES)

OLIGOSACCHARIDES	STARCH POLYSACCHARIDES	POLYSACCHARIDES
(3 to 20 molecule)	(20+ molecule)	(20+ molecule)
Partially digestible	Digestible	Indigestible.
Dextrins/Maltodextrins	Amylose	Cellulose/ Hemicellulose
Fructo-oligosaccharides	Amylopectin	Pectins Gums
Raffinose	Glucose polymers	Mucilages
Stachyose		Algal polysaccharides
Verbascose		Beta-glucans/Fructans

(Modified from Benardot, D. Advanced Sports Nutrition, 2006)

The maximum glucose that can be stored in skeletal muscle and liver has been determined, and is known as the glycogen saturation point. The liver has a maximum storage capacity of approximately 90 gm or 360 kcal. Skeletal muscle can store approximately 350 gm or 1400 kcal. The larger the muscle mass, the larger the glycogen storage, but also the higher the potential use of glucose.

To sustain a blood sugar level within such a narrow range, the liver is continuously releasing glucose either via the breakdown of glycogen stores, or through synthesis the novo. Sixty percent of the glucose released is directly coming from stored glycogen. The other 40% comes from glucose synthesized in the liver from lactate, pyruvate, amino acids (glutamine & alanine) and fat (glycerol). See figure 5.

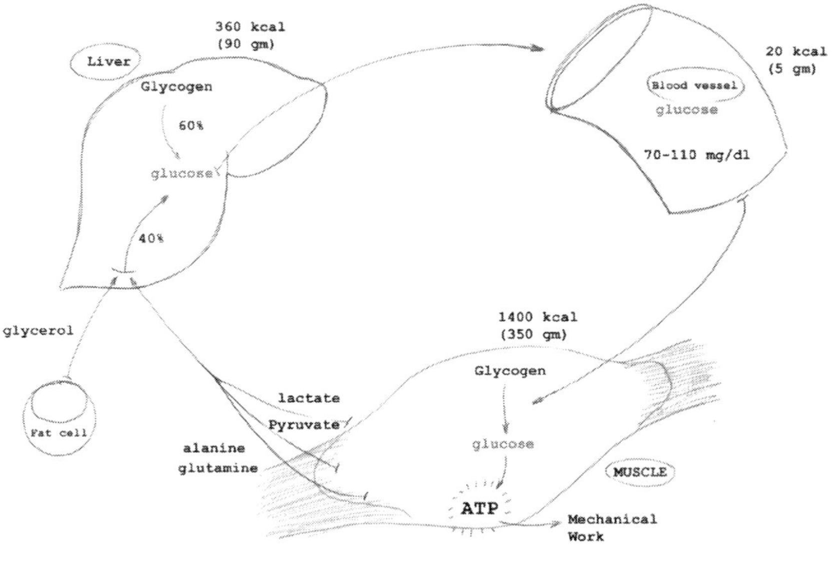

Fig. 5 Glycogen storage and release

This blood glucose needs to be transferred to the working cells and this is all facilitated by insulin, a hormone produced and released by special cells in the pancreas known as beta-cells. The stimulus for insulin secretion is high blood glucose which is actually what happens when we consume carbohydrates. The smaller the carbohydrate molecules (simple sugars) the faster and higher the blood glucose levels, hence the insulin levels. The larger the carbohydrate molecules (complex carbohydrates) the slower the digestion and absorption processes, therefore, the slower and lower the glucose levels, hence the insulin levels. The relative ease or difficulty by which certain carbohydrates yield a fast or slow blood sugar level, hence, insulin response, is what led to what is commonly known as the Glycemic Index of carbohydrates. We will come back to this later.

When blood glucose falls, as occurs in between meals or during exercise, another hormone, glucagon, is released by the alpha cells of the pancreas, which will increase blood glucose by breaking down glycogen stores from the liver (glycogenolysis) and by increasing the synthesis of glycogen from non-glucose sources (amino acids – alanine), a process known as gluconeogenesis.

If food supply (carbohydrate) is inadequate and exercise continues or the exercise intensity is higher, two hormones, epinephrine and cortisol, both released by the adrenal gland, come in handy to increase blood glucose levels. Epinephrine (adrenaline) increases glycogenolysis (glucose released from the breakdown of liver glycogen) and cortisol increases glyconeogenesis (protein breakdown, that yields alanine which is converted to glycogen in the liver). Therefore, if we consume the right carbohydrates during exercise, we can control the release of epinephrine and cortisol and their deleterious physiologic effects which include muscle protein breakdown and liver glycogen depletion. Let's not forget about insulin. Insulin has anabolic effects (muscle building) facilitating aminoacid inflow into the muscle cell. Aminoacids are the building blocks of muscle and connective tissue. Insulin also facilitates the uptake of triglycerides by fat cells, which as we learned, will be used as fuel during low to moderate to moderately high exercise intensities.

Now that glucose is finally in the muscle cell, it is here where our energy metabolic systems (aerobic and anaerobic) execute their mission. Both the aerobic and anaerobic metabolic systems generate ATP. The anaerobic pathway will do so in the absence of oxygen and this takes place inside the cell, outside the mitochondria. The aerobic pathway takes place inside the mitochondria, and as its name implies, in the presence of oxygen. See figure 6.

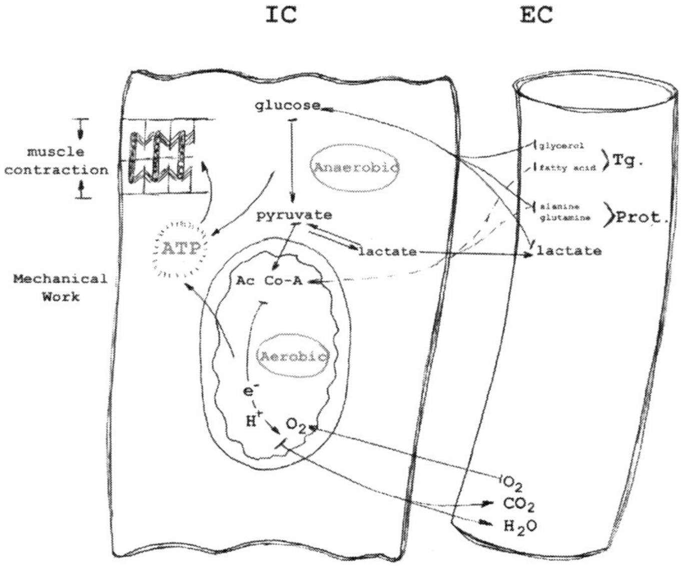

Fig. 6 The Glycolytic (Anaerobic) and the tri-carboxilic (Aerobic) metabolic pathways

As we can see, glucose undergoes a series of biochemical changes that end up in a molecule known as pyruvate. This first biochemical pathway in the absence of oxygen is known as the glycolytic pathway. During this glycolytic pathway, ATP is being generated. Pyruvate is continuously generating lactate, which is constantly being recycled, thereby avoiding its accumulation. Pyruvate is also continuously generating Acetyl Co-A, which in the presence of oxygen will proceed inside the mitochondria into a second biochemical pathway known as the tri-carboxylic acid pathway (Krebs cycle). The release of hydrogen ions (H+) and electrons (e-) are carried down into the electron transport system, ultimately to undergo oxidative phosphorylation (oxygen as a substrate) yielding its final waste products, carbon dioxide (CO_2) and water (H_2O). During this reduction/oxidation process ATP is generated. These processes inside the mitochondrium led to its popular name, the "RedOx" factory of the cell. As exercise intensity increase, the cardiopulmonary and circulatory systems fall short in providing the oxygen required to efficiently run the intramitochondrial oxidative phosphorylation pathway. Pyruvate can no longer run into the Acetyl Co-A pathway. More lactate is generated and the recycling system is overwhelmed, leading to lactate accumulation and from here a series of biochemical reactions that ultimately affect mechanical work and muscle contraction, manifested clinically as extreme muscle fatigue and exhaustion.

When we consume food we want those with great nutritional value and which carry the least amount of "contaminants." We also want enjoyable treats. When we exercise we also want food with great nutritional value and high in fuel. In general, carbohydrates are high in fuel, but like anything else, they are not created equal and, in fact, some provide "high octane – clean fuel" while others provide "low octane – contaminated fuel." Then, there are those which provide some "diluted fuel." The "low octane-contaminated fuel" foods are no good for you and in fact some could be potentially harmful. In today's market there are a lot of them. I will give you examples, but I will not spend too much time on them. We want variety where we can choose from and we also want fresh foods, those that will provide you with additional nutrients, vitamins and minerals, in addition to the main macronutrients (carbohydrates, protein, and fat). The way we store, process, and cook our foods, will either preserve or sometimes destroy and reduce their nutritional value. In general, most fresh, natural foods are "high octane – clean fuel." Fresh vegetables, legumes, fruits, nuts, grains, and lean cuts of meat, chicken and fish have great nutritional value. Within these groups there are some high in fuel but lower in nutritional value while others have high nutritional value that are low in fuel. The Nutrition Facts Label from the FDA's Center for Food and Safety and Applied Nutrition (CFSAN) provides important information for the public, athletes included. The label displays the percentage of the recommended daily value (%DV) of the nutrient per serving size based on a 2000-calorie a day diet. Needless to say, people who exercise, and even more so, athletes, require high caloric intake, sometimes in excess of 4,000 to 6,000 calories a day. The energy expenditure can be very high and prolonged, sometimes in excess of up to 20 calories per minute during events like the Tour de France or the World "Iron Man" Championships. Use the nutrition facts label for what it is worth. Use it as a reference and choose high %DV for vitamins, calcium, iron, fiber, and low %DV for fats, which should not comprise more than 25-30% of the total caloric intake. You should pay particular attention and limit the content of saturated fat and avoid altogether "trans-fats/hydrogenated fats." The poly-unsaturated and monounsaturated fats are good fats and should be an integral part of the athlete's nutrition program. I will be talking more about fats later on.

Quite frankly, I don't believe people know or even care about this nutrition facts label unless you have a medical condition that might force you to know and learn about your disease and your diet. Even under those circumstances, I don't believe people either know or basically do not care.

We could live healthier lifestyles and avoid many of today's major medical problems if we would only watch our waistlines, exercise, and eat balanced and nutritious diets.

"HIGH OCTANE/HIGH FUEL" CARBOHYDRATES

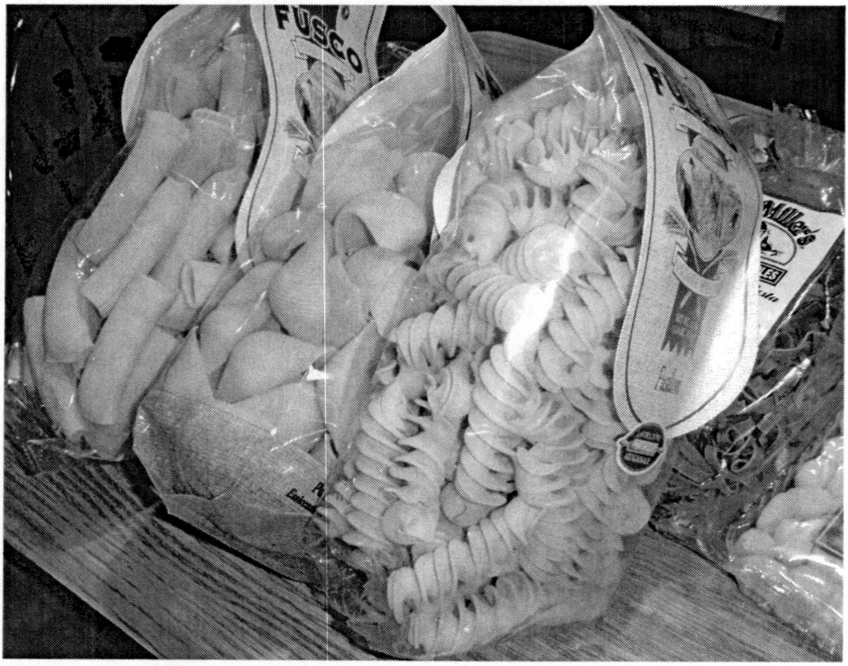

Athletes and nutritionists know pasta is one of the most important fuel sources and still retains its high nutritional value.

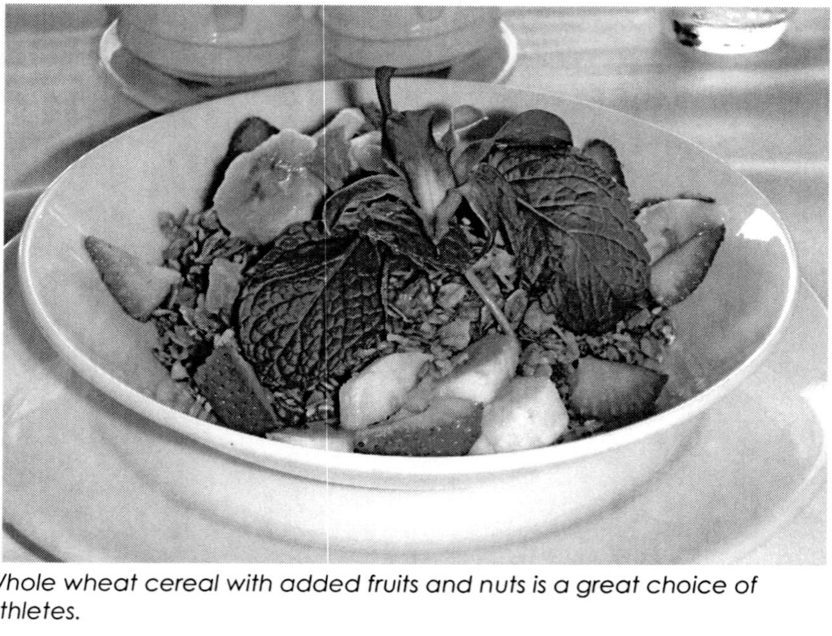

Whole wheat cereal with added fruits and nuts is a great choice of athletes.

Grains, cereals and pastas

This group includes wheat, rye, barley, corn, muesli, and oats which are amongst the most commonly known and available. Some possibly less common or unfamiliar grains include kasha, quinoa, bulgur, and others. In addition to the high carbohydrate content, they have a high nutritional value. They provide fiber which has multiple benefits including the increased bulk and softening of stool which can help the more than two million patients that seek a physician's visit a year for constipation alone. It reduces common GI problems like diverticulosis (weakening and pouching of the walls of the large intestine), some studies suggest a reduction of some types of cancer (stomach, colon, and GB cancer), and clearly a positive impact on heart disease and diabetes mellitus (delays the absorption of glucose, helps with bad cholesterol, there is some indication that it prevents the formation of small clots that can trigger heart attacks and strokes). They also contain some antioxidants (vitamin E), phyto-estrogens that can protect against some cancers and cholesterol-clogged arteries. The bran-layer of some grains contains essential minerals like magnesium, manganese, selenium, and copper which have very important physiologic roles. During the processing stage of most grains the hulls are removed which protected the grains while attached to the plant. The bran and germ are gone and with them lots of fiber, minerals, saturated fats, and antioxidants.

When shopping for grains and foods derived from them (bread, pasta, bagels, etc.) most authorities recommend, even if they have been ground into flour, to look for "whole grains," like whole wheat, cracked wheat and basically whole grain cereals. Pasta, which is big in most American households and restaurants, is essentially made from flour, water and salt. There are several whole-grain varieties of pasta, which in the case of some athletes as we know, has become a very important, if not the most important fuel and still retains its high nutritional value. Brown rice has a high nutrient value, higher than white rice, and for the athlete switching from one to the other, from time to time, is not a bad idea. Variety adds to your nutrition contentment as long as we don't forget the "high octane – high fuel" stuff.

Unquestionably, compliance is the biggest factor in the success of any nutrition or exercise program and in the case of most athletic individuals they tend to stick "with the program" because it becomes a lifestyle for them. Their friendships, vacation time, etc., is their world and they live accordingly.

Low "carb" diets don't work for athletes. The reason low carb or high carb, low fat or high fat, high protein, do not work for people, or they do so most of the time temporarily, is because these diets are not part of their lifestyles. You have to match your diet with the lifestyle you lead.

Cereals that have been cracked, split, or puffed, are the best choice for athletes and these include oats and muesli, though whole grain corn and pearl barley are also great. Some of these cereals are commercially available with added nuts, dried fruits, almonds, walnuts, raisins, dates, and some seeds like sesame seeds or flaxseed. You can also add them to your favorite cereal and, thereby, increase the nutrient value, and calorie intake based on your energy expenditure needs.

Going back to the glycemic index of foods and how they affect your blood sugar and insulin response, it is important to make clear that all tested foods (specifically containing carbohydrates) was limited and restricted to just a few volunteer individuals (approx. 8 to 10).

This was a slow and painstaking effort to test the same individuals several times to different foods having tested that individual first to a "pure glucose load." We have to remember that we all process food differently. We respond to glucose a little different than the volunteer individuals from where these numbers were obtained. The way we actually consume food in the real world is very different than in the laboratory where these individuals were tested which, again, was one food item at a time. Most of the initial attention to the glycemic index came from its use in diabetics and low-carbohydrate dieters. For this population, it is true that some foods containing "carbs" might be better than others when lack of insulin or insulin resistance is a problem. The glycemic index might be more accurate when taking a single food snack than it is when eating a "real meal," with multiple foods to be processed. However, I will stick to my goal here which is to illustrate how some foods are excellent to obtain quick energy by increasing your sugar levels rather fast, while other foods are more suited for long training sessions or for replenishing glycogen stores after exercise.

Glucose has a glycemic index of 100 in virtually all people. The glycemic index of a particular food is obtained by dividing the blood sugar response to the test food (i.e., potato or banana) by the response to pure glucose in the same individual. Here is a partial list of foods with high, moderate, or low glycemic indexes. Please refer to table 4.

TABLE 4 GLYCEMIC INDEX OF COMMONLY EATEN FOODS

CLASSIFICATION	FOOD	SERVING SIZE	CARBOHYDRATE (gm)	GLYCEMIC INDEX
HIGH (>70)	English muffin	1 muffin	11	77
	Whole wheat bread	1 slice	13	71
	White bread	1 slice	14	70
	Cheerios	1 cup	20	74
	Potatoes – mashed	1 cup	20	74
	Shredded wheat	2 biscuits	20	75
	Jelly beans	1 ounce	28	78
	Grape nuts	½ cup	41	71
	Cornflakes	1 cup	48	81
	Pancakes	2 – six inch	56	83
	Baked potato (with skin)	1 cup	51	85
	Baked sweet potato (with skin)	1 cup	48	81
	Honey			73
	Waffles (Aunt Jemima)			>80
	Bagel			>80
	Sports drinks		Variable depending on brand and volume	>80

	Bran muffin			>80
	Orange juice (concentrate)			>80
	Ocean Spray Cranberry juice cocktail			>80
MODERATE (55-70)	Coca-Cola	12 oz	39	63
	Cranberry juice	1 cup	36	68
	White rice	5 oz	36	64
	Snickers bar	1 bar (2 oz)	32	68
	Raisin Bran	1 cup	35	61
	Oatmeal (rolled oats)	1 cup	22	58
	Ice cream	½ cup	13	61
	Sugar, table	1 tsp	10	68
	Brown rice (steamed)			
	Oranges, strawberries, apples			
	Soy milk, low-fat			
	PowerBar Performance Bar			

LOW (<55)	Banana (ripe-brown tips)	1 medium	25	51
	Orange juice (not concentrate)	1 cup	23	52
	Strawberry jam	1 tbsp	20	51
	Pasta	1 cup	47	42
	Pizza Hut – Super Supreme Pizza	2 slices	24	36
	All-Bran Kellogg's	½ cup	21	42
	Baked beans	1 cup	15	48
	Skim milk	1 cup	13	32
	Pumpernickel (dark rye bread)	1 slice	12	41
	Chocolate			
	Carrots			
	Lentils			
	Chick peas			
	Peanuts, cashews			
	Ice cream – premium ultra-chocolate 15% fat			

Some reference sources for this list of glycemic index foods do not necessarily include the serving size, or the carbohydrate content, hence the blanks left in the table. The list, however, is helpful and practical and there are nutrition books with extensive lists that might suit your needs and preferences.

"HIGH OCTANE-MODERATELY HIGH TO MODERATELY LOW – TO – LOW FUEL CARBOHYDRATES"

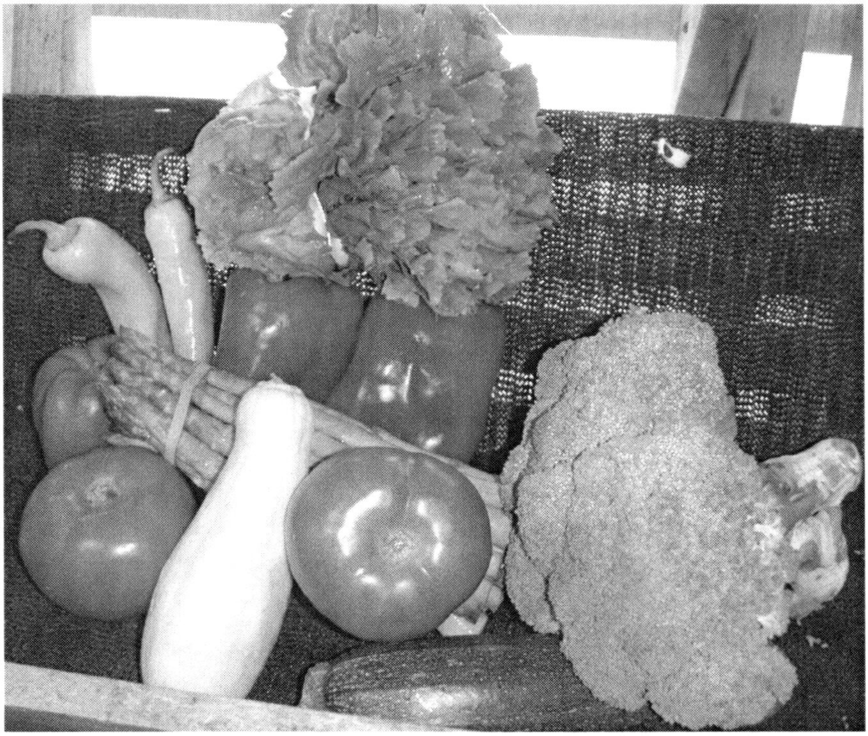

The more vibrant and intense the color of both fruits and vegetables, the higher the content of phytochemicals.

Vegetables and fruits

Believe it or not, even the United States Supreme Court System back in the late 1800's ruled that tomatoes were a vegetable, not a fruit, based on a tax fine scandal on imported fruits and vegetables.

You can figure out the rest. "Eat your vegetables!" The saying goes, from generation to generation.

When it comes down to great nutritional value, these two lead the way. Some are a great source of carbohydrates like sweet potato and baked potato (with skin). Some, however, have very little fuel despite their tremendous nutritional value (spinach and lettuce). It has been quoted that the more vibrant and intense the color of both fruits and vegetables the higher the content of phytochemicals (literally chemicals made by plants), vitamins and minerals. They provide lots of essential elements and fiber. However, the vast majority of these phytochemicals have yet to be discovered, named, chemically characterized and biologically evaluated. To name just a few of the known phytonutrients, I will list them as follows:

1. Vitamins and minerals.
2. Plant hormones: Isoflavones and phytosterols.
3. Soluble and insoluble fiber.
4. Isothiocyanates, thiocyanats, indoles, and nitriles.
5. Protease inhibitors.
6. Salt containing compounds: Allicin and Diallyl Sulfate.
7. Limonene and coumarin.
8. Lycopene and lutein.
9. Carotenoids and beta-carotene.
10. Clearly many more to follow.

Some of the health benefits of a diet rich in fruits and vegetables are:

1. Lower chance of a heart attack or stroke.
2. Lower blood pressure.
3. Lower your cholesterol.
4. Gastrointestinal benefits on constipation, diverticulosis, and possibly preventing cancer.
5. Prevention of other types of cancer.
6. Improving vision, maybe preventing some forms of cataract and macular degeneration.

7. Preventing memory loss and thinking skills.
8. Weight control by inducing satiety.
9. Many more.

Sorry to disappoint you, but vitamin supplements in pills are actually no more than that. They, in fact, do not contain the very many phytochemicals found in fresh fruits and vegetables that yield the tremendous health benefits that I briefly discussed. It is conceivable that some of these phytonutrients interact with each other, targeting different cells and tissues in exact proportions and combinations. It is also possible that one chemical present in a fruit may be required by a chemical present in a legume to execute their beneficial biologic effect.

Don't get me wrong, vitamin supplements are very useful, particularly so when people's diets are inadequate in many essential foods or when people for one reason or another, have other health issues that might not allow their consumption or absorption. Athletes come in a variety and this is also true for foods. There are as many foods and recipes as there are people in this world. We should strive to provide athletes with whatever their needs are to maintain healthy, active, and hopefully athletic successful lives.

Based on the many phytonutrients that fruits and vegetables provide, some people have looked into "scoring systems" that would help determine which ones are better than others. The Center for Science in the Public Interest (CSPI) has done exactly that. The score system is higher if they contain at least seven of what they consider "important nutrients." I will give you some examples, though extensive listing and scoring systems are available through the "Nutrition Action Newsletter" or at www.spinet.org/nah/fanfruit.htm. Please see table 5.

Table 5 indicates different nutrients, scores, and actual phytonutrient content.

TABLE 5

		PHYTONUTRIENT	
VEGETABLE/FRUIT	SCORE	HIGH 20-100 %DV	ADEQUATE TO MODERATE 5-19 %DV
Baked sweet potato / guava	424/421	Both carotenoids, Vit C	Both K^+, fiber, folate
Spinach raw / watermelon	287/310	Both carotenoids/Vit K – Vit C	Folate, Vit C / K^+, fiber
Red pepper / grapefruit	261/263	Both carotenoids, Vit C	n/a / K^+, fiber, folate
Butternut squash / cantaloupe	176/200	Both carotenoids, Vit C	Fiber / K^+, folate
Asparagus / kiwi fruit	163/233	Vit K, folate / Vit C	Both carotenoids, fiber / Vit C, K^+, folate
Orange, strawberries, apricots	186/173/156	All Vit C – most folate	All K^+, fiber, most carotenoids
Baked potato (skin), Baked potato (no skin)	139/69	Vit C, Iron, K^+, fiber – Only Vit C	Folate – K^+, fiber

This listing just illustrates the collective "score" grouping of some of the many available and nutritious fruits and vegetables. For instance, avocado which is technically a fruit, is a great source of vitamin C, folate, potassium, fiber, and monounsaturated fatty acids, which as we will review, provide an excellent source of the "good fats," the "high octane – non-contaminated fuel." Also, some vegetables and fruits provide more carbohydrates than others. In general, vegetables/legumes provide more grams of carbohydrate per serving than fruits do. The grams per cup for baked potato (with skin), sweet potato (baked with skin), garbanzo beans, and white or yellow corn are 51, 48, 45, and 41 respectively. The grams per serving for raisins (a quarter of a cup packed), banana (1 large unit), pear (1 medium sized), and grapes are 33, 30, 25, and 24 respectively.

Finally, I will mention a word on fiber. Generally speaking, foods higher in fiber tend to have a lower glycemic index. Some athletes love them, however, some are more cautious, particularly so because they are a source of gas and distention and certainly not a good choice immediately prior to an athletic event. Fortunately nature has provided us with soluble and insoluble fiber. Soluble fiber creates a gummy, sticky, kind of carrier that traps some cholesterol rich substances in the intestine that, in fact, generate less gas and distention and in addition provide cardiovascular health benefits from the lowering of cholesterol. Insoluble fiber has benefits as well. Remember, they have a lower glycemic index, hence, with tremendous benefits for diabetic athletes, particularly avoiding high levels of sugars and triglycerides which pose a significant problem in this particular population. See table 6 for vegetable and fruit fiber sources.

TABLE 6 VEGETABLE/FRUITS – FIBER SOURCES

SOLUBLE FIBER	INSOLUBLE FIBER
Apples	Barley
Bananas	Beets
Barley	Brussels sprouts
Beans / legumes	Cabbage
Carrots	Cauliflower
Citrus fruits	Fruits and vegetables with skin
Oatbran, Oatmeal	Rice (except for white)
Peas	Turnips
Rice bran	Wheat bran
Strawberries	Wheat cereal
Sweet potatoes	Whole wheat breads

According to AMDR (Acceptable Macronutrient Distribution Range) 45-65% of the total caloric intake should be carbohydrate. On the nutrition facts label, the %DV for carbohydrate is based on a recommended intake of 60% of total caloric consumption. I believe these label recommendations are more suited for the general public than they are for the athlete. I would agree more with the CTS (Carmichaels' Training Systems) emphasis on grams per pound of body weight, such that from the foundation phase up to the specialization phase, the actual macronutrient percentages reflect the increased carbohydrate consumption by elite athlete's with some adjustments in protein and fat intake. What is clear is the fact that people who consistently exercise and definitely more so the athlete, require a higher percentage of carbohydrate than what is recommended by the AMDR.

II. LIPIDS (fats)

Lipids, more popularly known as fats, have been condemned as a nutrient for two reasons. First, is the increasing weight gain and obesity of the American public over the last 50 years and at least to some extent, all blamed on fat consumption. It is true that fat has more than twice the calories than either protein or carbohydrates. Though this has not been the only reason, but rather the overall increased caloric intake, all macronutrients included. The second reason is the conclusive and overwhelming association of "high" cholesterol and cardiovascular disease which is the number one cause of death of all industrialized countries. We will discuss this a little bit more later on.

The AMDR (Acceptable Macronutrient Distribution Range) recommends a daily fat intake of no greater than 20-35% of the total calorie intake. Only athletes who have massive energy expenditures or who need to maintain very high weights (i.e., linemen on football teams) or who need higher fat intake to compensate for lower caloric intake (i.e., athletes that need reduced carbohydrate intake), would benefit from this strategy. From experience in medicine and cardiovascular disease, and based on scientific literature, there is no reason to believe that more than 20-25% of total daily calories should be from fats. However, few Americans consume less than 35% of total calories from fat.

There are different types of fats, some of which are clearly unhealthy and some of which have clear health benefits. In fact, lipids are very important. They are basic structural components of all cell membranes and they are the basic structure of all sex hormones and corticosteroids. The lipo-soluble vitamins (vitamins A, D, E, and K) for instance, are delivered in a "fat package." Some fats need to be consumed due to the fact that our bodies are incapable of synthesizing them and these fats are called the essential fatty acids of which I will be talking more about as we go along.

Virtually every cell in the body can synthesize cholesterol and the body can also manufacture phospholipids, triglycerides, and other fat molecules. Cholesterol, oils, butter, and margarine are all fats, though all with different characteristics and molecular structure. Fats refer to lipids that are solid at room temperature and oils to those lipids that are liquid or semi-liquid at room temperature. The most commonly consumed form of lipid is the triglyceride, which chemically consist of a glycerol (3-carbon alcohol) molecule and three attached fatty acids. The glycerol component of the molecule is metabolized like a carbohydrate for energy. In fact, when two glycerol molecules in the liver are bonded together, a new molecule is manufactured and already known to you as glucose. Fatty acids are naturally bonded to glycerol (triglyceride) once they are stored (i.e., fat cells, liver or muscle), however, to fulfill their metabolic functions, they split from each other and each one separately goes to their specific metabolic pathways to execute their function (generate energy, form part of membranes, etc.). Like carbohydrates, lipids are carbon, hydrogen, and oxygen atoms glued together. In the case of fatty acids, some carbon atoms are fully saturated with hydrogen ions and thereby known as saturated fatty acids. If some of the carbon atoms are double bonded to other carbon atoms they are less saturated with hydrogen ions, hence, the name of nonsaturated fatty acids. Fatty acids with one double bond are known as monounsaturated fatty acids. If two or more double bonds are present, they are known as polyunsaturated fatty acids.

Some fatty acids are not synthesized by our body and need to be consumed with our diets. These fats are called "essential fatty acids." The essential fatty acids are two: Linoleic (Omega-6) and Linolenic (Omega-3) fatty acids. Both essential fatty acids are polyunsaturated and the term Omega-3 or Omega-6 refers to the site of attachment of the last double bond from the end of the carbon chain. Excellent sources of saturated fatty acids include fats of animal origin (meat, poultry, dairy, and to a lesser extent fish), palm kernel oil and coconut oil. Monounsaturated fats are in abundance in olive oil and canola oil, nuts (predominantly almonds, hazel nuts, peanuts, pecans, pistachios, and walnuts) and to a lesser extent, in animal fat. Vegetable oils are rich in polyunsaturated fatty acids (with the exception of olive oil which is 75% monounsaturated).

Finally, the polyunsaturated "essential" Omega-6 (linoleic) and Omega-3 (linolenic) fatty acids are in abundance in vegetables oils (corn, sunflower, peanut, canola) and oils of cold-water fish (salmon, white fish, trout, caviar, sword fish, sardines, and tuna) or shellfish (shrimp) respectively.

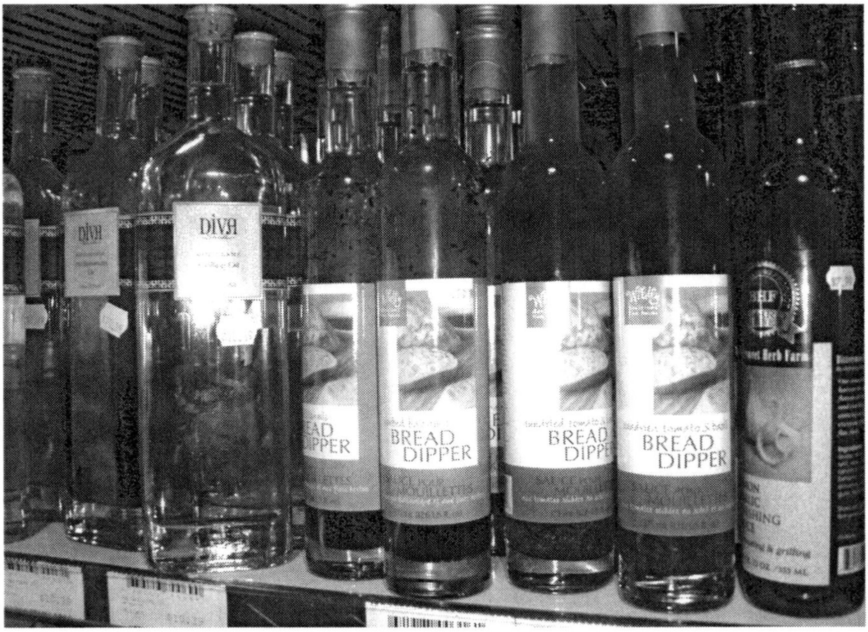

This excellent fat in liquid form, Olive Oil, is truly high octane - noncontaminated fuel.

Let me give you a word on lobster. When one is looking at a 3-ounce serving, the one nutrient that you get with lobster is protein. The total caloric value is 83 with 0.5g of total fat. The actual amount in grams of saturated, monounsaturated, polyunsaturated, Omega-3 and Omega-6 fatty acids are 0.09, 0.14, 0.08, 0.07, and 0.004 respectively. So, if you are looking to obtain the benefits of "good fats" from lobster, you are looking in the wrong place. On the other hand, if you are looking for protein, pleasure, fancy delicacy, and expense, then, here you hit the jackpot!

The AMDR for Omega-6 and Omega-3 fatty acids is 5 to 10 grams and .6 to 1.2 grams per day respectively. Because they are quite available and easily obtained, I don't believe most athletes have a problem meeting these requirements. Most athletes are highly motivated individuals and to a greater or lesser extent, they know what they are doing when it comes down to eating and food consumption.

There are three important messages that I would like to leave with you. There is an increase in heart disease with increasing saturated fat intake, it is also known that replacing saturated fats with unsaturated fats saves lives, and there is some connection of dietary fat with cancer.

Special highlights on Omega-3 fatty acids

There are there main types of Omega-3 fatty acids in our diets:

1. ALA (alpha-linolenic acid) – 18-carbon molecule "medium length chain."
2. EPA (eicosapentaenoic acid) – 20-carbon molecule "long length chain."
3. DHA (docosahexaenoic acid) – 22-carbon molecule "long length chain."

ALA is used mainly for energy. Food sources include a variety of vegetable oils and nuts, leafy vegetables and animal fats, especially from grass-fed animals. The body can transform it to EPA and DHA. EPA and DHA are structural components of cell membranes (i.e., the eye, brain, and sperm cells). They are part components of hormones that are involved in the contraction and relaxation of small blood vessels (arterioles), active components in the process of inflammation, blood clotting, amongst many others. They are very important modulators when it comes down to heart attacks and cardiac deaths. Different mechanisms appear to be responsible for their benefits which include: lowering the clotting tendencies of arteries clogged with cholesterol, which, as we know, appears to be the ultimate mechanistic event of a heart attack; preventing life-threatening erratic heart rhythms; improving the bad cholesterol and other particles in blood that contribute to "clogging" of the arteries, and limiting local inflammation, which contributes to the initiation, development, and ultimately the tear of the "plaque" that leads to a heart attack. I hope this message is clear.

The potential athletic benefits of Omega-3 fatty acids according to some authors include:

1. Reduce blood viscosity which increases oxygen and nutrient delivery.
2. Improve aerobic metabolism due to increase oxygen delivery.
3. Improve post exercise recovery time and anabolism due to the growth hormone's response to exercise, sleep, and hunger.
4. There is an anti-inflammatory component which leads to improved recovery time and decreased overall muscle fatigue.

According to some exercise physiology experts, the improved aerobic metabolism and the athlete's ability to effectively burn fat as an energy substrate appears to be one of the most important observations. The energy pooled in stored fat, even in the fittest and leanest athlete, ranges between 50,000 to 100,000 calories. I already discussed that you could theoretically bike 1,000 miles without having to stop to refuel. There is another 2,000 to 3,000 calories of triglycerides stored in muscle which appears to be readily available for energy needs. This IMTG (intramuscular triglyceride) is the first fuel to burn in the oxidative metabolic furnaces. How much time it takes to replenish the stores is unclear. What is clear is that maximal fat oxidation occurs at 65% of the individual's maximal oxygen consumption (65% of VO_2 max). As you recall, at higher workout intensities, the energy metabolic system depends more on the glycolytic anaerobic system and less in the aerobic oxidative system. At lower exercise intensities, the proportion of fat burned is higher when compared to higher exercise intensities and this should not be confused with the total amount burned, which is again higher, at higher exercise intensities. Keep in mind that if you are sitting down watching videos and football games, you are not going to burn fat and lose weight. The more you move the more you burn and if your exercise intensities are kept at 65% of your VO_2 max, you burn more fat and lose more weight.

Of real concern, are the "trans-fats" or "hydrogenated vegetable oils." As of 2006, the new nutrition facts label had to spell out the term "partially hydrogenated" or "vegetable shortening." These types of fats are particularly bad for the cardiovascular system. These fats raise the "bad cholesterol" in your blood and particularly the smaller "dense" LDL (low density lipoprotein) particles, which appear to have a higher tendency to deposit in the arterial walls. They also increase your triglycerides and lipoprotein (a), both of which have been linked to heart disease. They also lower the levels of HDL (high density lipoprotein) cholesterol, the "good cholesterol," which has beneficial effects as a "reverse transport molecule" of cholesterol from the arteries back to the liver. Basically it cleans the arteries of cholesterol.

When chemists mix some of the good polyunsaturated vegetable oil in the presence of hydrogen ions at high pressure heat, some of the hydrogen gets attached to the carbon backbone molecule and some of the double bonds are changed into single bonds. This is how hydrogenated fats, "trans-fats," were manufactured years ago. Here we ended up with a more saturated fat than an unsaturated fat and this is in part what led to some of the health issues that we're talking about. Let me give you some examples of very popular foods and the actual "trans-fats" content in grams per serving: Red Lobster "Admirals Feast" (1 serving) 22 grams, Long John Silvers "Fish and More" (1 serving) 14 grams, KFC "chicken pot pie" (1 serving) 8 grams, Burger King "French fries" (1 large) 5 grams, Dunkin Donuts "old fashion cake donut" (1) 6 grams.

I hope that current Federal rules will make these companies understand these issues and help eliminate, or at least substantially reduce the use of these hydrogenated fats in their cooking practices.

What about eggs?

Clearly egg consumption has declined over the last 50 years. When the link between "cholesterol" and cardiovascular disease became public, one of the most revered foods was actually almost vilified and condemned. Suffice to say, the extra 200mg of cholesterol a day provided in one egg is not going to "clog" your arteries. The fact of the matter is, eggs are very low in saturated fat and the nutritional value is outstanding, providing all essential and nonessential aminoacids, some polyunsaturated fats, complex B vitamins, folic acid, and vitamin D. What I see as a problem is the way people consume eggs. To give you an example, a standard breakfast on a weekend will include 2-3 eggs cooked in butter, with "fatty" cheese, bacon, and sausage. If you add to this, a muffin, which is rich in "trans-fats" and whole milk, there you have a perfect cardiovascular cocktail for future coronary events and strokes. Some people in fact have this routine 2-3 times a week. It is not a matter of whether they are going to run into a cardiovascular event, but when. On the other hand, "a healthy cocktail" would be one that includes one egg a day, maybe three to four days a week, cooked in canola or olive oil and add to this, "good grains," cereal, and fruit with skim milk and juice, and needless to say, this will give you enough protein, good carbohydrates and energy to be able to get on the treadmill or your bicycle and get a good exercise workout.

A word on dairy

From milk to yogurt, to cheese, to ice cream and butter, overall, dairy products are good for you with some exceptions. In addition to protein, these products are high in vitamins A, D, B2 (riboflavin), calcium, phosphorus, and good "cultures of bacteria" which are good for your intestine and digestion. Some products have more animal fat than others. A low-fat yogurt (fruit) – 8 oz serving, provides you with 232 calories, 2 grams of fat, 300mg of calcium, and 104 IU of vitamin A. On the other hand, a chocolate ice cream "Häagen-Dazs" – 8 oz serving, provides you with 540 calories, 18 grams of fat, 200mg of calcium, and 1000 IU of vitamin A. Butter and margarine are both rich in fat, however, butter is mostly "saturated" fat and margarine is mostly "polyunsaturated" fat. The problem with some of the margarine available is the fact that some have gone through the process of "hydrogenation," hence, their drawback. More and more companies are incorporating less and less "hydrogenation." Always read the labels, pick the ones with no "trans-fats" and as far as butter is concerned, use it sparingly or what I find as an excellent substitute is, "dip your bread" or "toast your bread" in olive oil. So go on, don't be shy, eat your healthy fats, but be aware of the good fats and the bad fats available in the market.

III. PROTEIN

There is a relative misconception on protein consumption amongst both endurance, but even more so power athletes. There is a belief that if they do not consume their "protein supplements," they will not perform optimally. This is not true for the individual who eats "plenty and healthy" for his gender, age, and level of physical activity and type of sport. Some athletes, however, do not fall in this category. They are eating on the run, their choices are either inadequate or insufficient, and this leads to an imbalance of supply and demand. Considering that 1 oz of meat provides approximately 7000 mg of aminoacids, and that the typical "protein-aminoacid" supplement provides somewhere between 500 to 1000mg, it certainly does not make too much sense. However, the reason we eat protein is solid. Proteins are the building blocks for cells, tissues, enzymes, and hormones that control metabolism and motion. Some of the protein's major functions include:

1. Enzyme formation responsible for many digestive and chemical processes.
2. The structural components of cells and tissues (heart, musculoskeletal system, liver, etc.)
3. Working proteins and hormones (Hemoglobin-oxygen transporter, Insulin-glucose metabolism, Serotonin-neurotransmitter, Actin and Myosin-muscle contraction).
4. Carrier proteins (transferrin-iron carrier, lipoproteins-fat carriers).
5. Immune system (antibodies-targeting foreign protein invaders, hence, fighting infections. Inflammatory chemical mediators helping with injury and repair).

6. Amphoteric molecules (regulating the acidity and alkalinity of blood environments).
7. Oncotic pressure properties (control of fluid volume and osmolality which maintains water balance both outside and inside the cells).
8. Energy (excess protein which becomes fat for storage and carbohydrate for gluconeogenesis-new glycogen from alanine and glutamine).

So what is a protein? Protein is a large molecule made up of smaller molecules named aminoacids. Aminoacids are bound together by what is known as the peptide bond. Here again, the backbone is a series of carbon, hydrogen, and oxygen atoms, but this time they have incorporated nitrogen, and in some cases, sulphur into their make-up. The aminoacid has an "amino group" bonded to the "carboxylic group." Some aminoacids are non-essential, meaning that they can be synthesized from other aminoacids. Some, however, must be obtained from the diet that we consume, hence, the name of essential-aminoacids. When we consume food, the protein is broken down into polypeptides, or smaller proteins, and these are broken down into aminoacids which are then absorbed and transported throughout the body. The different cells, tissues, and organs pick them up and, based on the cells "brain," the DNA, decide when and what to use, using their highly sophisticated RNA messenger molecules. As we have seen, the human body is the most beautiful expression of intelligence: the universe in its microversion, a microverse if you will.

Proteins undergo different biochemical transformations, two, which are very important and known as transamination and deamination. With transamination, the nitrogen of one aminoacid is used to synthesize a new aminoacid. With deamination, the nitrogen, "amino group," of a specific aminoacid is removed and converted to ammonia ($NH_2 \rightarrow NH_3$) which is toxic to the body. The liver converts ammonia to urea, which is eliminated with the urine. The rest of the carbon backbone of the aminoacids can be stored as fat or carbohydrate or burned for energy.

If you eat too much protein, this is "extra" work and an extra load to the body, that either will be stored as fat or will require more water to be eliminated through the urine as urea. There is also the potential to increase the elimination of calcium and all of these effects are very dangerous, particularly in people with specific types of kidney problems or kidney impairment.

PROTEIN REQUIREMENTS AND PHYSICAL ACTIVITY

The recommended daily protein intake in the general population has been estimated to be between 12 and 15% of the total caloric intake. The regular individual requires .8 grams per kilogram of protein a day, however, in the athlete, due to a greater lean mass, the need for tissue repair, the small amounts of protein lost in the urine, especially with high intensity exercise, and the small amount (10-15%) burned during high intensity physical activity, this requirement increases from 1.2 to 1.7 grams per kilogram of body weight.

Some of the essential aminoacids, known as branched-chain aminoacids (BCAA) – leucine, isoleucine, and valine, can be easily broken down and more readily used for energy. As we have seen, some other aminoacids (alanine and glutamine) need to be recycled to glycogen, ketones, or fatty acids, before they end up in the metabolic energy furnaces. As you recall, creatine phosphate (Cr P) and ATP, are immediately available to the anaerobic alactic metabolic system. Creatine can be made from other aminoacids (glycine, arginine, and methionine) in the liver, pancreas, and kidneys. One gram of creatine can also be obtained from large portions of red meat (approximately 250 grams). A 150-pound athlete will require approximately 2 grams of creatine and this is where our body's wisdom comes in and synthesizes what is actually required.

Carnitine is a protein responsible for transporting fatty acids into the mitochondria to generate ATP. Aerobic and endurance training increase both the number of mitochondria and the synthesis and storage of carnitine. Carnitine is made up from the aminoacids lysine and methionine. These co-factors appear to be responsible for the increased rates of aerobic energy production, derived from burning fat at higher exercise intensity.

Protein Sources

Protein can be obtained from both animal and plant sources. Nature has provided for everybody, including the vegetarian. Protein sources are considered complete when they contain all of the "essential aminoacids" to meet the metabolic needs. Protein sources are considered incomplete if at least one essential aminoacid is missing. Vegetables do not qualify as "complete," except for one, soybean.

Animal sources

Sources of "complete" protein include meat, poultry, fish, eggs, and dairy. It is here where you can choose the lean cut to avoid the "bonus" of saturated fat. Red meat also provides you with zinc, (more readily absorbed from meat sources than vegetable sources), iron, a fundamental component of the hemoglobin molecule, the most important oxygen carrier, and B-complex vitamins. Some cuts contain more saturated fat than others. T-bone steak (beef), beef hamburgers and ribs contain higher saturated fat than chicken breast, beef or pork sirloin, or top-round beef. Chicken and turkey contain a somewhat lower amount of zinc and iron than red meat. Fish and seafood are above and beyond the rest of protein animal sources; "High Octane!" In addition, you have the tremendous health benefits from unsaturated fatty acids, particularly the Omega-6 and Omega-3 fatty acids.

There has been some concern regarding fish consumption and possible poisoning with mercury (Hg), a heavy metal, PCB's (polychlorinated biphenyls) and other contaminants. Currently the effects of mercury or PCB's are not clear. These contaminants are dangerous at the high doses you would expect with industrial accidents. The word is out there for young children and women of childbearing age or pregnant women, to be cautious and prudent, particularly with some types of fish, including: shark, swordfish, king mackerel, and tile fish (sometimes called golden snapper or golden bass). The FDA also advises limiting the consumption of canned albacore (white tuna), however, not so much light tuna.

Plant sources

Again, with the exception of soybean, plant sources are considered "incomplete." Grains and cereal, vegetables (legumes) and particularly nuts and seeds, are good sources of protein. As we have seen, they also contain phytonutrients, fiber, folates, magnesium, monounsaturated and polyunsaturated fats, and multiple vitamins.

I would like to focus my attention now on the vegetarian athlete. I will emphasize plant sources of protein, particularly so nuts and soybean. Here is a list of non-animal sources of protein: It is highly recommended to combine seeds and nuts, cereals and legumes, in the same meal to some extent, to obtain a complete distribution of the essential aminoacids. Please refer to table 7.

TABLE 7 PLANT SOURCES OF PROTEIN

SOURCE	***EXAMPLES***
Nuts and seeds	Almonds
	Hazelnuts
	Peanuts
	Pecans
	Pistachios
	Walnuts
	Brazil nuts
	Cashews
	Macadamias
	Pine nuts
	Flaxseed
	Sunflower seeds
Grains and cereals	Granola
	Oatmeal
	Muesli
	All Bran
	Raisin Bran
	Corn
	Whole wheat
	Brown rice
	Barley
	Bulgur
	Pasta

Vegetables/legumes	Soybean Dried beans Dried peas Lentils Split peas White beans Kidney beans Black beans Pinto beans Chick peas

In general cereal, legumes, and vegetables are good sources of valine, threonine, phenylalanine, and leucine. Corn and other cereal grains are good sources of methionine and tryptophan, but poor in isoleucine and lysine. Legumes, on the other hand, are poor in tryptophan and methionine, however, they are good sources of isoleucine and lysine. Hence, combining these foods will ensure the athlete with a good and complete supply of all essential aminoacids.

Why nuts?

Depending on the study that you look at, some report a 30 to 50% lower risk of dying from atherosclerotic cardiovascular disease or heart attack with nut consumption. They appear to ameliorate the risks of developing type II diabetes mellitus (sugar diabetes) and gallstone disease. So, how do they help the heart and prevent cardiovascular disease? The unsaturated fatty acids improve LDL cholesterol and HDL cholesterol. The Omega-3, ALA, prevents clot formation and potentially deadly erratic heart rhythms. Nuts provide arginine, a non-essential aminoacid, which will be incorporated into a molecule known as nitric oxide, which leads to relaxation of constricted blood vessels, thereby improving blood flow. In addition, it makes platelets (blood cell particles that participate in clotting) less sticky, hence, lowering the clotting potential. Nuts are also a great source of energy, vitamin E, folic acid, potassium, fiber, and other phytonutrients.

Soy.

Is soy the answer for vegetarians? I think it is a great substitute for animal protein. It provides all of the "essential aminoacids" and clearly doesn't have the added saturated fat and cholesterol of animal fat and, in addition, has phytonutrients, some of which have clear health benefits. When compared to the animal protein counterparts, it has overall less protein, vitamin B2, calcium, and little vitamin A and vitamin D. However, there are many fortified brands out there that make these nutrients and vitamins more readily available. In fact, some brands may have more added calories than natural soy. It is probable that the effects on cholesterol and heart disease are in fact a reality. The FDA relies heavily on an article in the New England Journal of Medicine published some years ago, to approve the claim on the label that: "foods containing 6.25g of soy per serving and low in saturated fat may reduce the risk of heart disease." However, other claimed benefits are less well proven. These include some beneficial effects on memory loss, protection against breast, prostate, and other types of cancer, and postmenopausal symptoms. For every study claiming the pros, there is one claiming the cons. It is not my intention to discuss them here, but when you read one or the other, they sound pretty convincing. I personally do not believe that an isolated study or studies are the final word. Humans have been consuming soybean for centuries, even before we were living here in the Western Hemisphere. I think that what we have really learned in the last 100 years is that excess consumption, obesity, and physical inactivity has led to a very unhealthy lifestyle, that claims more lives than the combined next ten causes of death in the United States alone. I am referring to cardiovascular disease.

IV. FLUIDS

Ever since mankind stepped into outer space, the main objective has been a "search for life." Life, as we know it, is not possible without water. Water is life. We, human beings, are 55 to 75% water. This is the estimated percentage of a person's total body weight. Approximately 65% of the body's total water is inside the cells (intracellular) and the other 35% is outside the cells (extracellular). The higher the fat content of an individual the lower the percentage of water weight. The average female is approximately 50-55% water weight. Lean, muscular athletes are 70% water weight. Approximately 93% of blood is essentially water and the rest are cells, molecules, and minerals.

The heart is continuously pumping blood to the working muscles. Blood delivers oxygen, nutrients, hormones, and many different molecules that are necessary for optimal exercise performance and at the same time, it removes carbon dioxide, lactate, and other molecules for their disposal or their recycling metabolic pathways. This volume is kept within a relatively narrow range thanks to the perfect orchestration of baroreceptors (volume-pressure receptors), osmoreceptors (particles in solution), antidiuretic hormone (ADH), and aldosterone (adrenal gland hormone). Blood volume is affected by the concentration of sodium (Na^+), the main extracellular electrolyte, and other molecules like glucose and protein. The molecules and electrolytes are dissolved in blood. The concentration of these molecules will determine the osmolality (osmotic pressure) of blood. This osmolality is critical because it will determine the amount of water inside and outside the cells. When the osmolality in blood is too high, either due to excess salt or loss of fluid, the intracellular fluid pours out in an attempt to compensate and keep this osmotic pressure within a normal range. If the osmolality is too low, either due to low salt or excess fluid, this water will be disposed of via the kidneys or transferred into the cells. These osmoreceptors are located in a specialized part of the brain called the hypothalamus. When these osmoreceptors detect a high plasma osmolality, they activate the pituitary gland, ADH is released, which will then activate the kidney to retain water. This water retention tends to correct the highly concentrated blood. On the other hand, when the osmolality is too low, the hypothalamus inhibits the production and release of ADH, hence, increasing free water clearance by increasing water in the urine. Aldosterone is a hormone released by the adrenal gland in response to both low sodium and low blood volume. Aldosterone activates the kidney to reabsorb sodium (Na^+), which increases its concentration in blood. The increased sodium concentration retains water, hence, increasing blood volume. It is important to know that the main electrolytes in sweat, plasma, and the intracellular compartment are found in different concentrations for very specific and unique reasons, some of which will be reviewed shortly. Please refer to table 8.

TABLE 8 ELECTROLYTE CONCENTRATION IN THE INTRACELLULAR COMPARTMENT, PLASMA AND SWEAT (in mmol/liter)

	IC FLUID	PLASMA	SWEAT
Sodium (Na^+)	10	130-155	20-80
Potassium (K^+)	150	3.2-5.5	4-8
Calcium (Ca^{++})	0.1-0.3 to 1 μM/lt	2.1-2.9	0-1
Magnesium (Mg^{++})	15	.7-1.5	< .2
Chloride (Cl^-)	8	96-110	20-60
Bicarbonate (HCO_3^-)	10	23-28	0-35
Phosphate (PO_4^-)	65	0.7-1.6	0.1-0.2

Exercise generates heat. Energy metabolism is inefficient, meaning that somewhere between 25 to 30% of food energy is converted to mechanical work and the remaining 70 to 75% is converted into heat. This heat production, needs quick dissipation, otherwise it will continue to build up and lead to very serious complications including heat exhaustion, heat stroke, and death. It has been estimated that body temperature can increase at a rate of 1° F every five minutes, which means that, within one hour, a real threat to human survival is conceivable. The upper limit temperature rise is up to 110° F (43.3° C) after which death can occur. Our bodies can dissipate heat through sweat at a rate of approximately 1 milliliter per 0.5 kcal of heat production. Intense exercise, which can generate up to 900 kcal of excess heat over a one hour period, would lead to approximately 2 to 3 liters of water loss through sweat. This is especially true on hot humid days when sweating can be profuse. Virtually 85% of heat dissipation is achieved through evaporation (sweating) and radiation (vasodilatation-increasing blood flow to the skin). The remaining 15% of heat loss is through conduction and convection.

Thirst perception is considered a delayed physiologic response. Thirst becomes manifest with a rise in plasma osmolality somewhere between 2 to 3%, which approximates to a 1.5 to 2 liter water loss. Hence, thirst is a poor and delayed indicator of fluid needs. A reduction of almost 10% of blood volume is required to induce the thirst response, making this system even a less responsive mechanism for fluid replacement. The bottom line is that we should not allow thirst to happen before athletes start consuming fluids. Water consumption and replacement should become a conscientious routine prior to, during, and after exercise.

It is known that dehydration, by as little as a loss of 2% of body weight, will lead to impaired performance, and, losses in excess of 5% of body weight will impair exercise capacity by about 30%. Keep in mind that a negative nutrient balance can lead to significant impairment in exercise performance however, significant water loss can lead to life threatening conditions like severe dehydration, shock, heat exhaustion, or heat stroke, and actually death. A reasonable and practical method to estimate water loss and how much fluid you need includes:

1. Weigh yourself just before and immediately after training with no clothing (write down weight in pounds).
2. Monitor volume with fluids consumed during training.
3. Fluid loss = pre training weight – post training weight.

The actual calculation of total water loss should include the volume of fluids consumed during training. One liter of water weighs approximately 2 lbs. Sixteen ounces of fluid (1 pint) weighs approximately 1 pound. An additional 16 oz of fluid should be consumed for each 1-pound lost.

1 liter H_2O = 2 lbs

16 ounces H_2O = 1 lb

33.81 ounces H_2O = 1 liter

Example: Manni weighs 145 lbs prior to a 3 hour cycling workout. His weight immediately after exercise is 140 lbs. He consumed a total of 2 liters of hydration solution during this time period. Manni lost 3.5% of total body water (TBW).

145 lbs → 100%
140 lbs → X
X = 96.5% → {X = 3.5%} loss of TBW
Total H_2O loss = Net H_2O deficit + H_2O consumed
1 liter → 2 lbs
X liter → 5 lbs
Net H_2O deficit {x = 2.5 liters} (80 oz)
H_2O consumed = 2.0 liter (64 oz)
Total H_2O loss = 4.5 liters

Fluid replacement (FR) per pound lost → 16 oz
FR = 80 oz
1 liter → 33.81 oz
X liter → 80.0 oz {X = 2.4 liter} Rounding to 2.5 liter

For the next three-hour cycling workout or competition Manni should consume approximately 4.5 liters (approximately 145 ounces). This means, he needs to drink approximately 8 oz every 10 minutes to virtually replace all fluid loss, assuming no significant changes in perspiration, ambient temperature or humidity. The actual goal during workout or competition is to lose no more than 2% of total body weight regardless of the length of the event. The athlete should aim to consume no less than 80% of his water loss. It is of most importance to maintain an adequate blood volume. A lower blood volume due to excess water loss or lack of fluid replacement or both will lead to several physiologic responses including:

1. Lower stroke volume.
2. Lower cardiac output.
3. Increased heart rate.
4. Increased core body temperature.
5. Decreased skin blood flow (compromising heat dissipation).
6. Decreased muscle blood flow (compromising muscle glycogen use).

7. Increases of adrenalin and cortisol.
8. Increased or decreased osmolality and plasma sodium, depending on sodium losses in sweat.

Many investigators, in fact, consider blood volume (hydration status) the primary indicator of whether an athlete would be able to maintain a high performance during workout or competition.

In general, fluids are seen on a day in and day out basis, as a compliment to a meal, to make it easier to swallow solid food and to calm thirst, but truthfully, fluids should be regarded, especially by athletes, the same way nutrients are approached. Over and over, fluid imbalances are the most common cause of exercise underperformance and, clearly, the one thing that can be potentially life threatening. In sports, there are several factors that can affect water balance and increase water losses:

1. Increase duration and increase intensity of exercise.
2. Increase ambient temperature and increase humidity.
3. High altitude and especially so, in cold weather (air moisture).
4. Large body surface area (evaporating surface area).
5. Higher conditioning and training status (higher heat dissipation through evaporation – sweat).
6. Diets high in protein and sodium.
7. Increased hydration status (better hydration – higher sweat potential).
8. Clothing (some fabric might reduce cooling efficiency and increase a higher sweat rate).

However, the two main factors that will determine fluid intake are thirst and the taste and temperature of the hydrating solution. We will get back to this topic in part C of this book.

There are several fluid-related clinical conditions that I would like to touch upon, which are seen either very frequently or very occasionally, but which need very specific attention and sometimes even medical intervention. These fluid-related conditions include:

1. Dehydration.
2. Heat cramps.
3. Heat exhaustion.
4. Heat stroke.

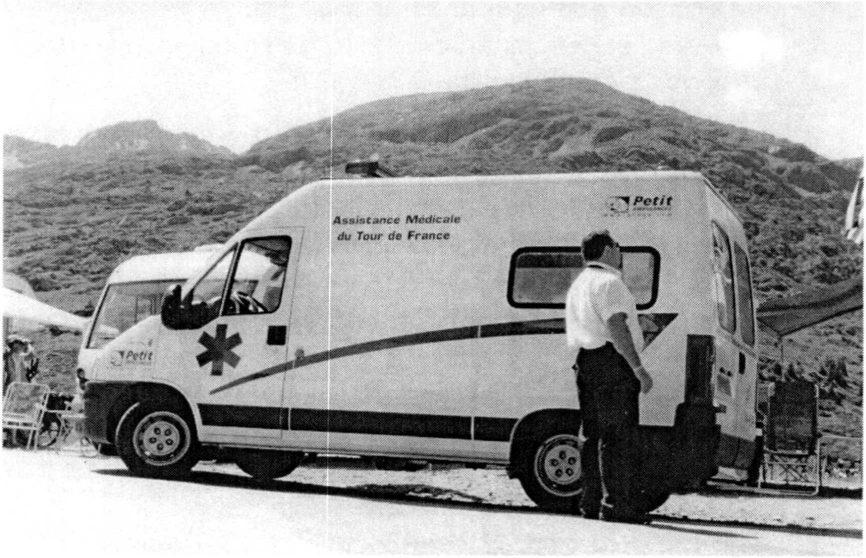

Prompt medical assistance in the athletic field is a must in any sporting event.

1. ***Dehydration*** – By definition dehydration means suboptimal body water. Impaired performance results from a 2% loss of body weight in water. Water losses in excess of 5% of body weight will impair performance by as much as 30%. The two most common causes of dehydration in athletes include inadequate fluid replacement and high sweat rates, and most of the time it is a combination of both. The four most common recognizable signs or symptoms of dehydration include:

- Thirst
- Inappropriate increase in heart rate.
- Decreased urine volume.
- Small concentrated urine (dark yellow).

There are different types and degrees of dehydration, but for the purpose of this book and practicality, to correct this water imbalance and deficit, the athlete needs fluids and electrolytes (Na^+, Cl^-, Mg^{++} and K^+). The athlete should drink plenty of a cold, tasteful hydrating solution that contains some sugar (glucose, sucrose, fructose, and maltodextrin) or a combination of sugars with small amounts of sodium and potassium. Solutions that contain between 6 and 8% of carbohydrate and salt are very well tolerated and intestinal absorption is faster. The rate of fluid replacement should be somewhere between 0.5 liters to 2 to 3 liters per hour, obviously depending on the severity of the dehydration. Some athletes might require intravenous hydration when they cannot tolerate oral intake, especially during the first hour or couple of hours after competition. After initial parenteral hydration, the athlete might spontaneously ask for a drink which is always a good sign. At that point oral hydration should be continued. Again, importantly, the athlete and coach should keep record of his weight prior to and after a training workout or competition whenever possible. Once thirst is corrected and urine volume increases (clear urine), most likely the heart rate will drop within a physiologic range. At this point adequate nutrition and additional hydration should resume.

2. ***Heat Cramps*** **–** Most athletes might have experienced spontaneous pain from muscle contractions of the legs and thighs, and even on rare occasions, spasms of the abdominal wall, shoulder, and neck. This is usually the result of severe dehydration and electrolyte imbalance. It appears most commonly in athletes who sweat profusely and who also have higher than normal electrolyte losses (Na^+, K^+, Ca^{++}, Mg^{++}). These individuals usually report very "salty tasting" sweat and sweat that "stings" the eyes. They notice visible "chalky," powdery salt on the face, arms, legs, and clothing during and after exercise. These are athletes who carry a history of "cramping," usually they sweat profusely early into physical activity, do not consume enough fluids and tend to keep a sodium restricted diet. Heat cramps are also more commonly seen with increased environmental temperature and humidity.

It is recommended that at the first sign of muscle twitching or cramping, athletes should consume at least ½ liter (16 oz) of a sports drink that contains electrolytes, particularly Na^+. Some of these athletes may have been consuming large volumes of hypotonic fluids or just plain water. This leads to hyponatremia (low sodium in blood). After the first 0.5 liters, the individual should resume sodium

– supplemented sports drinks at rates of at least 4 oz every five minutes for the remainder of the athletic event. Hopefully cramping will subside, otherwise, the athletic event can come to a halt. Prevention is a better approach. Hydration prior to the sports event and continuous steady intake of glucose and electrolyte containing drinks will prevent this embarrassing athletic mishap. There are commercial products available that can be added to the sports drink or can be taken as a pill (which will need to be chewed and grounded) and swallowed with the hydrating solutions.

3. ***Heat Exhaustion*** – This condition is recognized by a feeling of extreme fatigue and faintness, weakness, and a cold, clammy skin with a weak pulse pressure. There is none or minimal sweat and the athlete may display a tendency to faint, in and out of a semiconscious state. There is significant volume depletion and inadequate blood flow to the brain and kidneys with an increase of core body temperature.

Once recognized, the athlete should be cooled promptly with cooling blankets and cool wet towels or wet ice-cold cloths. If there is a low blood pressure with inappropriate tachycardia and poor conscious status, oral hydration should not be attempted. Under these circumstances, aggressive parenteral hydration is mandatory using normal isotonic saline solution or similar solutions with electrolytes like Ringer's lactate. The athlete should not resume his training or competition endeavor. Once the athlete's mental status is clear, fully awake and alert, oral hydration may be attempted, starting with sips of cool water and, if tolerated, move on to glucose and salt supplemented hydrating solutions (sports drinks).

4. ***Heat Stroke*** – By definition this condition is a thermo-regulatory failure with elevation in core body temperature and elevation of the hypothalamic set point.

Heat stroke has been recognized as a thermo-regulatory failure in a warm and/or humid environment in association with or without exertion. This condition needs immediate recognition and treatment, otherwise it can be fatal. The core body temperature is usually above 105° F (40.5° C), the skin is hot and dry, pulse is fast and damped and mentation is poor (many times unconscious). Not infrequently there are signs of dehydration and some individuals may have used over-the-counter antihistamines (with anticholinergic side effects) or prescription of psychotropic drugs or use of illicit drugs (amphetamines, cocaine, alcohol, and many more) that may exacerbate or precipitate exertional heat stroke.

The victim needs immediate cooling and first responders should call for an ambulance or whatever services are available in the athletic field (clinics or first-aid tents). Parenteral hydration is mandatory and should be continued with the cooling interventions until return to full consciousness. Subsequently oral hydration can be started.

What is a hydration solution and are sports beverages better than water?

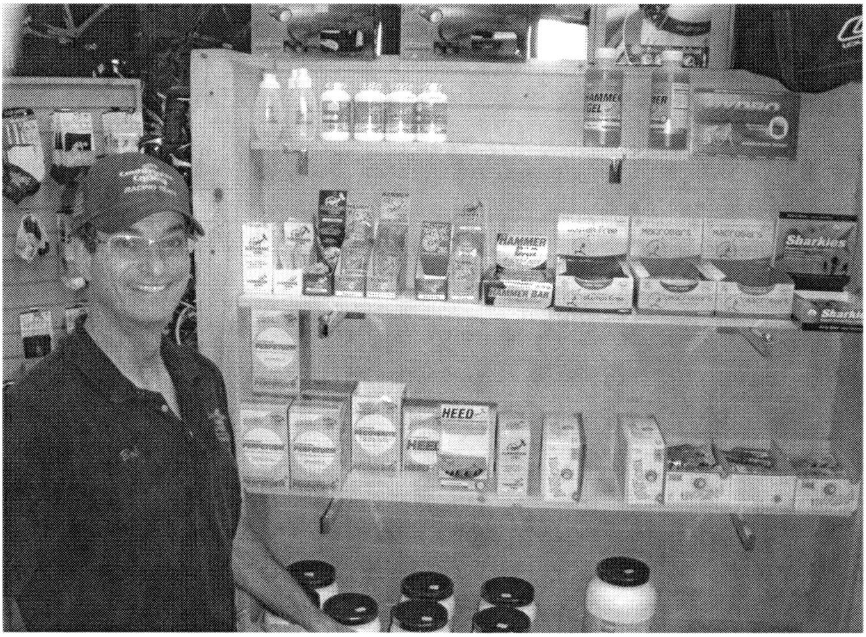

Sports drinks with multiple labels - Performance, recovery, replacement drinks (electrolytes, carbohydrates, protein, etc.) Courtesy of Robert Kramer, Countryside Cycling, Edinboro, PA

Assuming the athlete is always making a conscientious effort to eat a balanced diet with plenty of "high octane-clean fuel," vitamins and minerals, athletic events lasting less than 30 minutes to an hour are for the most part well taken care of with just plain water for hydration. However, under certain circumstances and especially so, for intense one-hour or longer sporting events, where you anticipate high sweating rates, some individuals achieve better hydration with solutions containing some sugar and electrolytes. Sports drinks containing sugar and electrolytes do improve performance and recovery and lead the athlete to better drinking habits. The market has exploded with a wide array of sports drinks ranging from electrolyte – replacement drinks, carbohydrate – replacement drinks, to protein and energy drinks. Like athletes, not all sports drinks are created equal and there is a great variety out there to choose from.

Sports drinks have different types and concentration of sugars and electrolytes, each trying to achieve the same goals:

1. Stimulate the drive to drink.
2. Deliver energy to the working muscles.
3. Supply electrolyte replacement.
4. Accelerate fluid and electrolyte absorption by facilitating gastric emptying.
5. Maintaining optimal hydration, hence an optimal blood volume.
6. Heat dissipation by preservation of skin blood flow through optimal hydration.

Several factors will determine the athlete's drive to drink. It is different having a glass of cold water at home on a warm summer day than a relatively warm sip of water after 2-3 hours on a bicycle. It is well known amongst athletes that food and drink taste differently before or after exercise than during training or competition. However, taste, texture, temperature, odor, and color of hydration solutions do make a difference and can stimulate the drive to drink. Highly concentrated beverages can taste too sweet, too thick or sticky, and can even feel "too heavy," upsetting to your stomach.

Sports drinks should feel smooth, slightly citrus flavored, refreshing, and slightly sweetened. These characteristics stimulate the drive to drink and if properly balanced, will accelerate fluid and electrolyte absorption. This is what most athletes like anyway.

Optimal concentration of carbohydrate in fluid will determine the solutions osmolality and thereby, the gastric emptying time and absorption rate. Studies have shown that the most effective drinks are those with 6 to 8% carbohydrate concentrations, whereas drinks with higher concentrations are less well tolerated and gastric emptying and absorption rates are lower. Most drinks today contain combinations of glucose, sucrose, fructose, and maltodextrin and, on an isocaloric basis, simple sugars (i.e., glucose) have slightly longer gastric emptying times than an oligosaccharide like maltodextrin. Studies have also shown that small amounts of sodium can stimulate drinking and to some extent, maintain the osmotic pressure and prevent severe dehydration (low plasma sodium) during prolonged exercise events, particularly so in individuals with very high sweating rates and sodium losses. Most sports drinks also contain small amounts of potassium, magnesium, trace elements, and more recently adding protein seems to have some probable benefits.

In a position statement on fluid and sodium replacement in sporting events lasting more than one hour, the American College of Sports Medicine guidelines recommend a sodium intake that ranges from 0.5 to 0.7g/l of fluid (21-30mmol/l) to 0.25-0.5g/hr for people susceptible to the risks of hyponatremia during ultra endurance events. Gatorade, a rather popular sports drink, will provide 0.33 to 0.41g, when ingested at a rate of 750ml to 1 liter/hr respectively. Table 9 is an abbreviated list of some popular sports drinks available in the market.

TABLE 9 LIST OF SPORTS AND RECOVERY DRINKS

- Accelerade
- All Sport
- Carboflex
- Cytomax
- Endurox R_4
- Enervit
- EFS
- Gatorade
- Optygen
- Orange juice
- Power-Ade
- Power-Bar
- Smartfuel
- Sustained Energy
- Ultima
- Ultra Fuel
- Water
- Sodas

For detailed information regarding carbohydrate content and electrolyte concentration, consider internet search or direct product label information.

PowerBar Endurance and PowerBar Performance Recovery drinks have a carbohydrate composition entirely from maltodextrin, dextrose, and fructose. The carbohydrate concentration ranges between 7 and 8.5% and they also contain 160 to 250mg of sodium respectively.

Beverages containing mainly fructose cause more gastrointestinal distress and maltodextrins are less sweet than sucrose or fructose. Some athletes have developed a high tolerance to higher carbohydrate concentrations without necessarily having significant intestinal distress or discomfort.

It is important to mention that standard sports drinks (10-25mmol/l of sodium and 35mmol/l of potassium) may not address the replacement of large electrolyte losses during and after exercise. Significant sodium losses through profuse sweating can present a real challenge when attempting to restore the salt (i.e. – 8 to 10 L sweat loss with a 60-70mmol/L concentration). Under these circumstances, food intake becomes very important due to the high Na^+ content of "real food" and the possibility of using the salt shaker. Specific recommendations regarding training and recovery nutrition and hydration will be addressed in part C of this book.

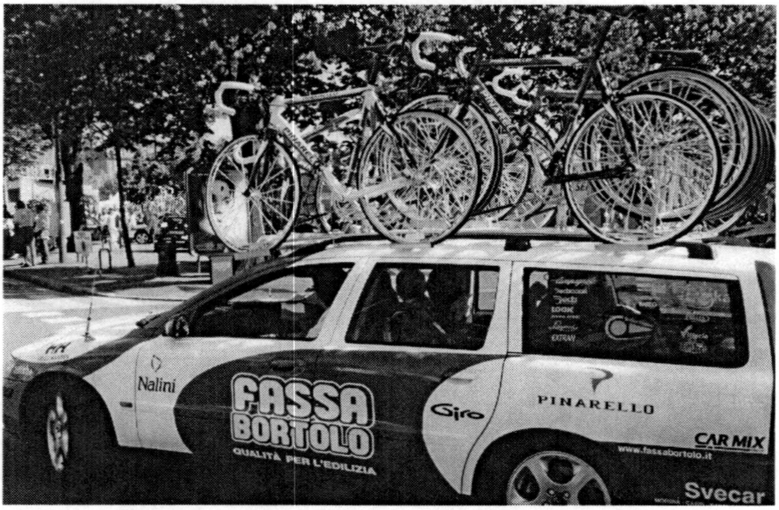

Support vehicles transport not only the tools of the trade and Director Sportifs, but also hydration and nutrition for the athlete.

V. VITAMINS AND MINERALS

Also known as micronutrients, vitamins and minerals are essential for life. Fortunately, a well balanced diet will provide, for the most part, all micronutrients in an otherwise healthy individual.

Vitamins are organic compounds required in very small amounts and, based on the relative solubility are classified as fat-soluble or water-soluble. Minerals are inorganic elements found naturally on earth and work either independently, (i.e., sodium – maintaining water homeostasis) or jointly with other organic nutrients (i.e., vitamin D and calcium – bone homeostasis or vitamin B12 and iron – hemoglobin oxygen transport). Based on daily requirements, they are classified as macrominerals (greater than 100mg/day) and microminerals or trace elements (less than 10mg/day).

In one way or another and to a lesser or greater extent, some of the most important effects of vitamins and minerals on body functions related to athletic training and performance include:

1. Co-factors and activators of the different energy metabolic systems.
2. Central nervous system function and impulse transmission.
3. Muscle contraction and relaxation.
4. Hemoglobin synthesis and oxygen carrying capacity.
5. Water homeostasis and plasma osmolality.
6. Maintenance of the relative acidity or alkalinity of blood and tissues.
7. Immune system.
8. Antioxidant function.
9. Bone metabolism.

Please refer to tables 10 and 11.

TABLE 10 SUMMARY OF THE MOST IMPORTANT EFFECTS OF VITAMINS ON BODY FUNCTIONS RELATED TO ATHLETIC TRAINING AND PERFORMANCE

	Co-Factor and Activators of energy metabolic systems	***Nervous Function Muscle Contraction***	***Hemoglobin synthesis***	***Immune function***	***Anti-oxidant function***	***Bone metabolism***	***Blood coagulation***
Thiamin (B1)	X	X					
Riboflavin (B2)	X	X					
Vitamin B6	X	X	X	X			
Vitamin B12		X	X				
Folic Acid		X	X				
Niacin	X	X					
Pantothenic Acid	X						
Biotin	X						
Vitamin C				X	X		
Vitamin A		X		X	X		
Vitamin D						X	
Vitamin E				X	X		
Vitamin K						X	X

Adapted from Burke, L., Deakin, V., Clinical Sports Nutrition, 2006

TABLE 11 SUMMARY OF THE MOST IMPORTANT EFFECTS OF MINERALS ON BODY FUNCTIONS RELATED TO ATHLETIC TRAINING AND PERFORMANCE

	Co-Factor and Activators of energy metabolic systems	***Nervous Function Muscle Contraction***	***Hemoglobin synthesis***	***Immune function***	***Anti-oxidant function***	***Bone metabolism***	***Water Homeostasis***	***Acidity Alkalinity***	***GI function***
Sodium (Na^+)		X					X		
Potassium (K^+)		X							
Calcium (Ca^{++})		X				X			
Magnesium (Mg^{++})	X	X		X		X			
Bicarbonate (HCO_3^-)							X	X	X
Phosphate (PO_4^-)	X	X				X		X	
Chloride (Cl^-)		X					X	X	X
Iron (Fe)	X		X		X				
Zinc (Zn)	X			X	X				
Copper (Cu)	X				X				
Chromium (Cr)	X								
Selenium (Se)					X				
Iodine (I)	X	X							
Manganese Mn)	X					X			

Adapted from Burke, L., Deakin, V., Clinical Sports Nutrition, 2006

In an otherwise healthy individual, most studies do not show any significant difference between athletes and non-athlete's indices of micronutrient status, nor have studies conclusively showed that micronutrient supplementation would increase physical performance. Studies do show, however, impaired performance when a deficiency is present, even if marginal. At CTS nutrition and diet habit questionnaires in athletes do show that the most neglected foods are fruits and vegetables. The FDA established the RDA (recommended daily allowances) for certain vitamins and minerals that are sufficient to meet the "minimal" requirement of nearly 98 to 100% of otherwise healthy individuals based on age and gender below which deficiency can occur. These are public health guidelines which have not been evaluated in athletes.

It is my opinion as a physician and athlete, and the opinion of experts in sports, that water and sodium are the most commonly encountered nutritional deficiencies in athletes. In clinical practice, after water and sodium, probably iron deficiency is next. In the older veteran athlete, particularly females, calcium deficiency prevails and is clinically detected early on using a special imaging technique known as bone density before actual complications of brittle bones can occur.

What about oxygen, oxidative stress, and antioxidants?

As we have seen, oxygen consumption can increase by 10 to 15 fold and in professional cyclists up to 20 to 25 fold. The oxygen flux to muscle during strenuous exercise can increase up to 200 fold. The incomplete reduction of oxygen yields reactive oxygen species, also known as free radicals. Our body is designed to counteract the potential oxidative damage to susceptible cells, cell membranes, enzymes, and structural proteins including DNA. These reactive oxygen species include superoxide (O_2^-), hydrogen peroxide (H_2O_2) and the hydroxyl radical (HO^-). Fortunately, we have a potent anti-oxidant system which includes some plasma proteins, bilirubin, uric acid, and the enzymes superoxide dismutase, glutathione peroxidase, catalase and others. This is known as the endogenous anti-oxidant system. Dietary products with anti-oxidant properties are known as the exogenous anti-oxidant system. Some of these anti-oxidants include vitamins E, C, carotenoids (beta-carotene), flavonoids, glutathione, co-enzyme Q10 and others. It is the belief amongst scientists in many fields and disciplines, that anti-oxidants keep the oxidative damage to a minimum by neutralizing these reactive oxygen species, minimizing the formation of new free radicals and probably repairing the oxidative damage of cells and tissues.

It has been postulated that aging, per se, is the body's response to oxidative stress during our lifetimes. My humble opinion is that this is anybody's educated guess. Many studies published in the most respectable scientific journals have demonstrated repeatedly the deleterious effects of oxidative stress in many organ systems and in many different unrelated clinical conditions ranging from the number one killer in the United States, atherosclerotic coronary artery disease to oxidative stress in the athlete, to aging.

I would like for you to stop and think here for a second. You are familiar with that grandpa who lived a normal life, was not an athlete, stayed active, ate well, and lived to be 92 years of age when he died of a heart attack. You are probably also familiar with the late Dr. Edmund Burke, PhD and world renowned exercise physiologist and recreational athlete who died suddenly at 50 years of age during a cycling training ride from a clogged artery that led to a heart attack. Both had been exposed to oxidative stress during their lifetimes. My understanding is that Dr. Burke was health conscious and knew well about anti-oxidants and their benefits.

If you say that oxidative stress killed them both, I can't disagree, however, if you say that it was not oxidative stress that caused their demise, I could not disagree either.

Oxidative stress is at the very core of the biochemical reactions that lead to cholesterol build up inside the arteries that supply the heart, the brain, and other vascular territories. Very important in-vitro and in-vivo studies have been performed in an attempt to understand oxidative stress and the potential benefits of both the endogenous and exogenous anti-oxidant systems. It is not the scope of this book to discuss these particular studies, however, very important clinical studies on exogenous anti-oxidants have failed to demonstrate conclusively a significant reduction in clinical events (i.e., heart attacks or strokes) when compared to placebo.

In the sports literature, as well, there is no conclusive data that would recommend the routine use of anti-oxidants (vitamin E, C, A). Athletes that have difficulty meeting their higher anti-oxidant requirements may benefit from supplementation. However, a diet that is high in anti-oxidants, will meet all the necessary requirements in athletes. The most neglected nutrients, fruits and vegetables, contain the most anti-oxidants. When it comes to healthy eating habits and diet counseling, this becomes one of the most challenging tasks to deal with. In the athlete, the problem is more related to a lack of understanding of human physiology and is the reason why some very accomplished professional athletes will go to the extreme of indulging in protein products, nutrient supplements including vitamins and some ergogenic aids such as pharmacologic (i.e., steroids, EPO) or physiologic aids (i.e., blood transfusions) which are banned by sports organizing committees and the International Olympic Committee. I will come back to this topic in our next section.

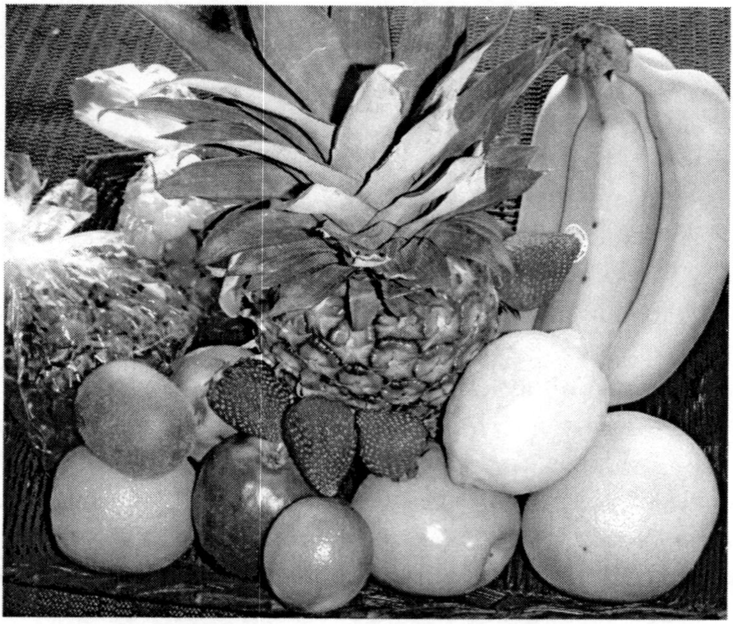

Phytonutrients found in fruits and vegetables are a great source of vitamins, minerals, soluble and insoluble fiber amongst others, just to name a few.

Tables 12 and 13 summarize the recommended intake of vitamins and minerals in athletes and food sources.

TABLE 12 RECOMMENDED INTAKE OF VITAMINS IN ATHLETES AND FOOD SOURCES

	DAILY RECOMMENDED DOSE	***BEST FOOD SOURCES***
Thiamin (B1)	1.5-3.0mg/day	Whole grain cereals, enriched grains, beans
Riboflavin (B2)	1.2mg per 1000 calories	Dairy, eggs, wholegrain cereals, enriched grains, dark green leafy vegetables
Vitamin B6	1.5-2.0mg/day	Meats, whole grain cereals, enriched cereals, eggs
Vitamin B12	2.4-2.5mg/day	Meat, fish, poultry, eggs, milk, cheese
Folic Acid	400mcg/day	Green leafy vegetables, oranges, bananas, beans and whole grain cereals
Niacin	14-20mg/day	Milk, eggs, turkey, chicken, whole grains, lean meat, fish, poultry, some grains
Pantothenic Acid	4-5mg/day	Abundant in all nutrients except for processed and refined foods
Biotin	30mcg/day	Egg yolks, legumes, dark green leafy vegetables
Vitamin C	200mg/day	Fresh fruits (citrus) and vegetables
Vitamin A (retinol)	700-900mcg/day	Cheese, egg yolks, fish liver oils, dark green and brightly pigmented fruits and vegetables
Vitamin D	5-15mcg/day	Fish liver oil, eggs, canned fish, milk (fortified), sunlight exposure
Vitamin E	15mg/day	Polyunsaturated and monounsaturated vegetable and cereal oils (olive, corn, soy)
Vitamin K	700-900mcg/day	Dark green leafy vegetables and vegetable oils

TABLE 13 RECOMMENDED INTAKE OF MINERALS AND FOOD SOURCES

	DAILY RECOMMENDED DOSE	***BEST FOOD SOURCES***
Sodium (Na^+)	1.5 to > 10gm/day (↑ sweat rates)	Table salt, salted foods, processed and canned foods
Potassium (K^+)	4.7gm/day or higher (↑ sweat rates)	Citrus fruits, potatoes, vegetables, milk, meat, fish, bananas
Calcium (Ca^{++})	1300-1500mg/day	Dairy, dark green leafy vegetables and legumes, Ca^{++} - fortified foods, soy milk
Magnesium (Mg^{++})	400-450mg/day	Dairy, meat, nuts, whole grains, fruits, dark green leafy vegetables
Phosphate (PO_4^-)	1250-1500mg/day	All high protein foods, whole grain products, carbonated beverages
Chloride (Cl^-)	2.3gm/day or higher gm/day (↑sweat rates)	Table salt, salted foods
Iron (Fe)	15-18mg/day	Meat, fish, poultry, shellfish, lesser amounts in legumes, dark green leafy vegetables, dried fruit
Zinc (Zn)	11-15mg/day	Meat, fish, poultry, shellfish, eggs, nuts, whole grain foods, vegetables
Copper (Cu)	900mcg/day	Meat, fish, poultry, shellfish, eggs, nuts, whole grain foods, bananas
Chromium (Cr)	30-35mg/day	Whole grain foods, nuts, legumes, cheese, mushrooms, Brewer's yeast
Selenium (Se)	50-55mcg/day	Meat, fish, seafood, whole grain foods, nuts
Iodine (I)	120-150mcg/day	Iodized salt, seafood
Manganese (Mn)	2.0-2.5mg/day	Whole grain foods, legumes, green leafy vegetables, bananas

VI. ERGOGENIC AIDS

By definition, an ergogenic aid refers to any nutritional, pharmacologic, psychologic, physical or mechanical aid that theoretically can improve athletic performance and possibly eliminate or ameliorate fatigue. From massage, hypnosis, music, to the use of anabolic steroids, blood transfusions, EPO (Erythropoietin), amphetamines, alcohol, and cocaine, athletes and coaches have tried numerous ways to achieve the athletes maximum potential and winning scores. The common practice of indulging in protein supplements, vitamins, minerals, and antioxidants is another commonly observed ergogenic approach. When considering an ergogenic intervention, you always have to ask yourself whether it is safe, effective and whether it is legal or not. Needless to say, the market is loaded with and selling ergogenic aids to anybody, especially those with little knowledge and big budgets. I have been around long enough to know better. I have to admit that probably one of the most desirable effects of most, however not all, ergogenic aids is the placebo effect. Most of the time there is little "hard" scientific evidence that there is a real performance-enhancing effect of these interventions. We live in a world of contradictions and ironies. Athletes spend long hours training, eating well balanced meals, getting close medical attention, however, some will fall into the "crazed, frenzy-indulging behavior," that will lead to potentially very serious consequences: From body function disruption such as anxiety, depression, irritability, liver disease, cardiovascular dysfunction, and myopathy (skeletal or cardiac muscle) to drug addiction and death. In addition, some will bring their careers to a halt either temporarily or permanently due to penalties imposed by sports organizing committees. Here is a partial list of substances that are or have been used by athletes and are considered illegal and/or banned by different sports organizing committees.

* Anabolic steroids (similar function to testosterone-male hormone).
* Amphetamines (central nervous system stimulants).
* Blood doping (autologous or homologous transfusions – self or type – matched donors
respectively).

* Beta-blockers and diuretics.
* Cocaine and other illicit drugs.
* Ephedrine and related substances.
* EPO (Erythropoietin).
* GHB and human growth hormone.
* Alcohol (ethanol – banned in shooting events).

The following list of products have been shown, in scientific trials, to provide performance benefit and are not considered illegal or banned from sports:

- Sports drinks.
- Liquid meal supplements.
- Sports bars and gels.
- Multivitamin/mineral supplements (including iron, calcium and anti-oxidants).
- Creatine? (creatine phosphate – (Cr P)-anaerobic alactic system).
- Glycerol? (3-Carbon water attractant – super hydration).
- Caffeine? (CNS stimulant and muscle relaxant).

Some products have no clear proof of performance benefit, however, are still used by many athletes. This group, I consider the "placebo, "budget drain" category:

* Amino acids
* Aspartates
* Bicarbonate
* Carnitine (L-carnitine)
* Co-Enzyme Q10 and Q12 – cytochrome C.
* Choline
* Chromium picolinate
* Ginseng
* Glutamine
* Glucosamine
* Glutamine
* Pyruvate
* Oxygen
* Oxygenated water
* Phosphates
* Phytosterols
* Tryptophan
* Vitamin B12 injections and other injectable forms of vitamins and iron
* Ribose (D-Ribose)
* Many more

I would like to finish this section with some comments on the "placebo" effect of most ergogenic aids. Let me make it clear that this is my own personal belief, however, based on many years of schooling, training, reading scientific literature, from physiology and biochemistry to philosophy and psychology to quantum physics.

Our brain is a rather complex organ designed to receive, process, and generate information. It is a universe of arranged molecules that obey the same laws of nature that operate the entire universe. The carbon, hydrogen, oxygen, and nitrogen atoms in the neuron (brain cell) or nerve sheaths are no different from these same atoms in a PowerBar or the nearest or farthest planet, star, or galaxy. Thoughts originate from quantum events at the subatomic level. These very finely tuned and elegant orchestrations of subatomic quantum events generate molecules (neuropeptides) and energy fields in pools of neurons which have been termed "neuronets." What we can detect with EEG's (electroencephalogram), scanners (CT, PET, MRI, etc.) and other technological gadgets are the finished products of these quantum events. These molecules and energy fields communicate with other neurons and "neuronets" to rearrange this molecular universe and there we have a thought, an image, a memory, a wish, a feeling, a creation, or without going to far, a voluntary muscle contraction that will become the 100-meter dash Olympic Gold Medalist or the seven-time winner of the Tour de France.

So we are what we believe we are. By definition, an ergogenic aid that does not produce a "true" physiologic effect is considered a "placebo" effect, because of some sort of psychological "boost." It has been said: "the placebo effect describes a favorable outcome arising simply from an individual's belief that they have received a beneficial treatment." If an athlete with a great genetic endowment does not believe he can become a champion, does not train or fuel properly, he will never become a champion. If this same individual trains properly and truly believes that he can become a champion, he will.

Lance Armstrong's fight with metastatic testicular cancer and his return to "stardom" is the result of a great genetic makeup and what Brad Kearns very succinctly calls the "success factors in action: positive attitude, clarity of purpose, specialized intelligence, and pure confidence." At the quantum level, these highly organized molecular events that define the structure and function of Lance Armstrong's heart, lungs, muscles, and energy metabolic systems will determine the high VO_2 max, lactate threshold, and power output of a champion.

However, the "success factors," are all quantum events in the mind of Lance Armstrong because he believed he would become a champion. So, it is the brain, the mind, which will determine some of the benefits of these ergogenic aids called "placebo," if you believe in them. The placebo alone will not make you a champion. The placebo alone might not work at all, after all!

Health

PART C: Training and Recovery Nutrition/Hydration

&

Fitness

I. PERIODIZATION AND NUTRITION – THE BASICS

Classic periodization refers to the weekly, monthly, and yearly cyclic variations in the "basic components" of training which include duration, volume, frequency, and intensity. The length of each training phase and desired training effects and ultimate results, will depend on the specific sport and the training-competition schedule. The dynamics of training-competition and the effects on the energy metabolic systems should be matched by the actual dynamics of nutrition (energy) and fluid intake.

In the professional athletic schedule, the training year is divided into three or four to five phases of varying durations. Different coaches and athletic programs have given these phases different names: Pre-season, competitive season, and off-season, is one example. At CTS (Carmichael Training Systems) they include the foundation, preparation, specialization, and transition periods. I will keep my training phases into the foundation, pre-competition (transition), pre-competition (taper), and recovery phases, that I very briefly discuss in my booklet, "The T-Zone Health and Fitness Cycling Training Program." Please be aware, that specific training schedule was designed for a 12-week training program, though the training phases in this section refer to a full-year training schedule. The weekly training unit is considered the shortest unit, which has been referred to as a micro-cycle. Two or more micro-cycles are considered a macro-cycle. Macro-cycles of different lengths are grouped units that constitute the actual training phases year round:

The foundation phase – the foundation phase can stretch from eight up to sixteen weeks, depending on the level of athletic competition and the specific sport. This phase requires long training sessions ranging from two to six hours at relatively low intensity. The focus is overloading the aerobic system and minimizing the contribution of the anaerobic lactic or alactic systems. Carbohydrates and fats are the basic fuels to maintain these prolonged-low intensity workouts. The aerobic metabolic system burns and even mixture of carbohydrates and fat. The 50/50 rule is a good way to remember the fuel-energy contributions in the foundation phase.

The pre-competition (transition) phase – The pre-competition (transition) phase or preparation period ranges from eight to twelve weeks, again, depending on the sport and athletic competition level. Training sessions are of intermediate length and volume and high-intensity, with maximum overloading of the aerobic system and active recruiting of the anaerobic system. Remember from our earlier discussions on the energy metabolic systems, as exercise intensity increases, you burn more carbohydrates than fat. The 70/30 rule is a good way to remember the fuel energy contributions during the pre-competition (transition) phase.

The pre-competition (taper) phase – The pre-competition (taper) phase or specialization period can be divided into early and late sub-phases. Usually it doesn't stretch out for more than four to eight weeks. During the early sub-phase, the training sessions are short to intermediate length, though at their most intense. Both the aerobic and anaerobic systems (lactic and alactic) are taxed maximally. Here, carbohydrates are burning faster and in great quantities. Also, there is tissue and muscle micro-injury that needs active and quick repair and the immune system is being maximally challenged. Protein intake takes over fats during this phase and adjustments need to be made. During the late sub-phase, there is a true tapering of two to three weeks of relatively short, low intensity training sessions during which, almost exclusively, the aerobic system is recruited with minimal, if any, contribution from the anaerobic lactic system. The liver and muscles have been trained to handle large glycogen loads and tissue and muscle repair are virtually completed.

The recovery phase – The recovery phase (transition period) is as important as the rest of the entire training program. It is time to rest and forget about the high demands on your physical body and psyche. Nonetheless, it is the most important period to maintain the basic aerobic fitness. Four to eight weeks of cross training in some other sport that you like, at low intensity, will keep that aerobic conditioning. Nutritional requirements will change to a less carbohydrate load and more protein intake, much needed in the repair of tissues and muscle and, replenishing of micro-nutrients.

TABLE 14 PERIODIZATION TRAINING AND ENERGY SYSTEMS

1-Year Training Schedule

PHASE	***FOUNDATION***	***PRE-COMPETITION (transition)***	***PRE-COMPETITION (taper)***		***COMPETITION***	***RECOVERY***
CYCLES – MACRO (months)	3-4 months	2-3 months	1-2 months		1-4 months	1-2 months
MICRO (week)			Early	Late		
TRAINING COMPONENTS	Long-high volume/low intensity	Sport specific intermediate length and volume/high intensity	Sport specific low to intermediate length and volume/very high intensity	Inter-mediate length/ low intensity	Maximum volume and intensity	Low to intermediate length and volume/low intensity
ENERGY (aerobic) SYSTEM (anaerobic) DYNAMICS	4+ (-)	3-4+ 1-2+	4+ 4+	3+ (-)	4+ 4+	2-3+ (-)
ENERGY SYSTEM FUEL REQUIREMENTS	Carb/fat 50/50	Carb/fat 70/30	Carb/Prot/Fat ↑ ↑ ↓		Carb/Prot/Fat ↑ ↑ ↑	Carb/Prot/Fat ↓ ↑ ↑

At CTS (Carmichael training systems) the recommended nutrient percentages of carbohydrate-protein-fat per body weight (in pounds) during the different training phases or periods is summarized in table 15.

TABLE 15

	BODY WEIGHT RANGE	**NUTRIENT PERCENTAGES (%)**		
	110-195 lbs	Carbohydrate	Protein	Fats
Foundation period	"	65	13	22
Preparation period	"	65	13	22
Specialization period	"	70	14	16
Transition period	"	60	18	22

(Adapted from Carmichael, C. Food for Fitness, 2004)

Excellent references are available that give a thorough and in-depth review on this subject.

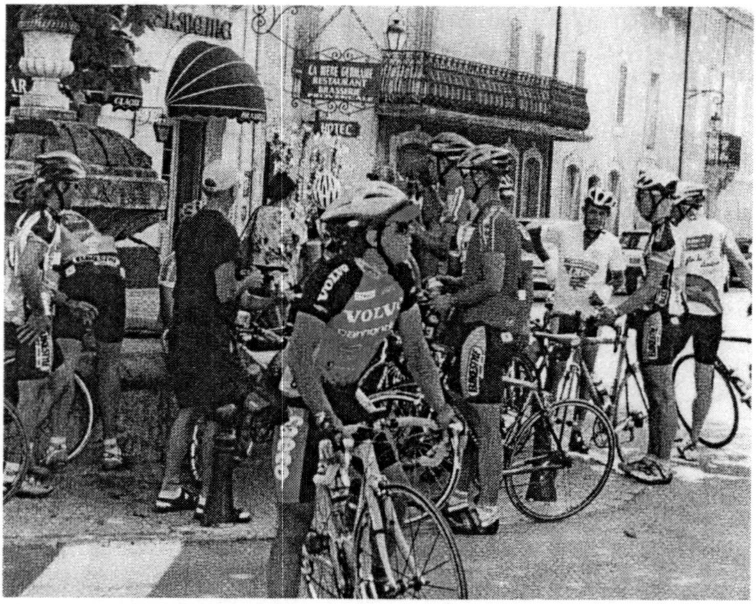

Tour de France ex-pros, Neil Stephens and Allan Peiper, insist that we fill up our water bottles and stay well hydrated. Tour de France 2002, Chateauneuf-du-Pape wine region.

II. NUTRITION / HYDRATION PRE-TRAINING – PRE-COMPETITION

Hydration goal: to get to the field or training session adequately hydrated (euhydrated) with normal plasma electrolyte levels for optimal athletic performance and nutrient delivery.

Nutrition goal: to get to the field or training session with normal muscle and liver glycogen stores that allows optimal energy substrate utilization and athletic performance.

Pre-hydrating with beverages (i.e., sports drinks) can or should be started two to four hours before the training or competition event. Remember that low volume and concentrated urine (dark urine with high osmolality and high specific gravity) is indicative of dehydration. The ACSM (American College of Sports Medicine) position stand on exercise and fluid replacement, published this year (2007), recommends starting hydration at least four hours before the exercise task, drinking somewhere between 5 to 7ml/kg of body weight and consider reloading with 3 to 5ml/kg body weight within two hours of the event if there is any indication of suboptimal hydration or dehydration. Sports drinks containing electrolytes, particularly sodium, will help stimulate thirst and retain the consumed fluids. This can also be accomplished by consuming salted meals or snacks (i.e., pretzels) and beverages.

Liver glycogen stores can deplete rapidly after an eight to ten hour overnight fast. Liver glycogen is responsible for the very timely and fine tuned release of glucose into the blood stream. For training and competition events lasting less than 60 to 90 minutes, there is no need, for the most part, for aggressive "carbo-loading," highly publicized over 35 to 40 years ago. However, today, carbo-loading still appears to have good use for training or competition events lasting more than 60 to 90 minutes.

A high-carbohydrate meal (0.5g/lb of body weight) consumed within 60 to 90 minutes prior to exercise, has shown to improve performance with minimal or no side effects. A large normal meal high in carbohydrates (2g/lb body weight) and good hydration is considered adequate if consumed at least four hours prior to exercise. Snacking on high and intermediate glycemic index foods and drinking carbohydrate-containing sports drinks every 10 to 15 minutes is an alternative, when approached within 60 to 90 minutes of the competition or training event. The most important thing to remember is that good eating and drinking habits will prevent fatigue and dehydration. Athletes should try different foods and feeding strategies before they get to the real competitive field. Experimentation the day of competition can be costly.

The "carbo-loading" concept has been around for many years and today, modifications to the original protocols are quite appropriately utilized for sporting events lasting more than 60 to 90 minutes.

The original Bergstrom et al (1967) protocol included both an early and a late phase. The early phase was a depletion phase with high-intensity exercise and low carbohydrate consumption. The later phase included a low-intensity and high-carbohydrate reloading phase. Both phases totaled seven days, which was rather cumbersome and potentially dangerous and today has been virtually abandoned.

Subsequently a modification by Sherman et al (1983) indicated a gradual exercise tapering with 50% carbohydrate consumption for two days followed by a reduced training load and a high carbohydrate diet. All too cumbersome and some athletes did not care for it due to interruptions or changes in their training, pre-competition schedule.

More recently Fairchild et al (2002) proposed a high-speed carbo-loading strategy that takes 24-hours, and reportedly, glycogen stores are comparable, if not higher, than in previous protocols. They indicate an ultra-hard and short workout (2-3 minutes) the day prior to competition, followed by a very high carbohydrate intake (90% of calories) over the next 24-hours.

In the resting, trained muscle, glycogen stores range somewhere between 100 to 120 mmol/kg/wet weight (ww). Muscle glycogen stores are rapidly restored after 24-hours of good rest and high carbohydrate consumption. Glycogen super-compensation or carbo-loading for endurance events lasting more than 90 minutes will elevate the muscle glycogen stores from 150 to 250 mmol/kg/ww.

Researchers have found that high pre-exercise muscle glycogen stores will postpone fatigue and extend the duration of steady-state exercise by approximately 20%, and improve performance or workload by 2 to 3%, hence, particularly suited for events such as marathons, triathlons, or cycling races and cross-country skiing events. Glycogen super-compensation can be achieved with 36 to 48 hours of rest and a carbohydrate intake of 10 to 12g/kg/day, which will contribute 75 to 85% of total calories. High glycemic index foods should be consumed at frequent intervals during the four hours after the last training session with plenty of fluids and electrolytes as has been previously described.

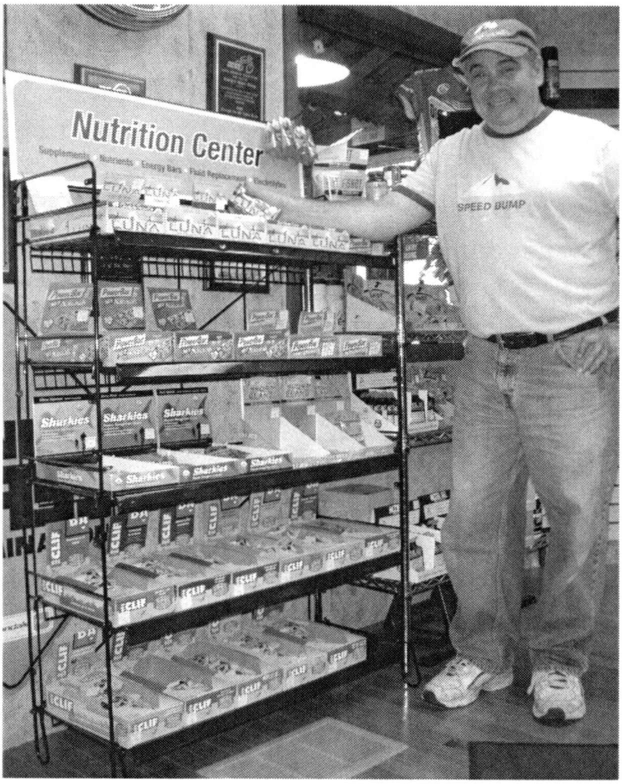

Nutrition packed in bars, gels, pills, etc. During competition they are a great source of energy. Courtesy of Pat Emigs, Emigs Bicycle Shop, Meadville, PA

III. NUTRITION / HYDRATION DURING TRAINING-COMPETITION

Hydration goal: to maintain adequate hydration status and electrolyte balance and to prevent excess water and electrolyte losses due to excess sweating rates, prolonged strenuous exercise and drinking opportunities. Losses of approximately 2% of TBW can hinder athletic performance by 10-15% and losses in excess of 5% of TBW by as much as 30% or, what is worse, can pose a threat to your health and life.

Nutrition goal: to maintain adequate glucose blood levels by preserving liver glycogen stores and avoiding depletion of muscle glycogen, which can lead to muscle fatigue and under-performance or, what is worse, compromise fuel supply to the brain leading to poor decision making, impairment of sports specific motor skills, all of which could potentially be a threat to your health and life.

When it comes down to hydration there is no magic formula for fluid replacement, however, the most sensible and practical recommendation is to monitor body weight and keep record of fluids consumed during training/competition as reviewed in section V, Part B of this book. Sweating rates can range from 0.4 liters to 2 liters per hour or higher depending on the intensity of exercise, weather conditions, training status, genetics, etc.

- *Events lasting less than 60 minutes* – these events, for the most part, do not tax body fluids and electrolytes as much as prolonged (greater than 1 hour and 3 to 6 hours or above) exercise. With time the cumulative effects are bigger and the mismatch between supply and demand increase. Also, energy stores are probably sufficient for most individuals assuming they have fueled properly as we have discussed previously. Plain water or a sports drink should suffice if taken at regular intervals during training/competition. Drinking somewhere between 16 ounces (0.5 liters) to approximately 54 ounces (2 liters) is usually sufficient. With adequate pre-event glycogen stores, the individual does not require high carbohydrate intake except for the carbohydrate supplied with the sports drinks.

- *Events lasting 1 to 3 hours* – the main concerns in these type of events include both fluid and carbohydrate replacement. These events are of low intensity when compared to less than 60 minute events. Athletes can better keep up with their fluid intake, though glycogen depletion can become a problem. According to the recommendations by the ACSM, carbohydrates should be ingested at a rate of 30-60g/hr (ACSM: 1996). Higher intakes, in excess of 60-70g/hr, will lead to gastrointestinal distress, delayed gastric emptying and will not result in increased carbohydrate utilization (Jeukendrup and Jentjens 2000). Here the athlete is "feeding on the run." Tour de France pros consume about half of the daily calorie intake during each day's cycling stage. Energy intake during running events is sometimes marginal due to intolerance to solid food by many of these athletes. Most of their energy supply is obtained from sports drinks and gels. Always read the labels! Try different sports drinks, energy gels, and bars. You can obtain 67g of carbohydrates from 0.5 liter of Boost (nutritional drink) if consumed within the hour. This will cover your energy requirements. Another way to meet your hourly requirements would be to drink 1 liter of Power Bar Endurance sports drink which will supply you with 61g of carbohydrates. Maybe you can't tolerate or need 1 liter per hour and would rather have some food or energy bars. Try three fig newtons (36g of carbohydrate) or one medium sized banana (30g of carbohydrate) or one Power Bar Performance Bar (45g of carbohydrate) and 0.5 liters of the same sports drink as above and you will get hydration and an additional 30g of carbohydrates.....and voila! 60g/hr recommendations are covered. Most sports bars will provide 40-50g of carbohydrates plus small amounts of protein (5 to 10g) and minimal amounts of fats and some vitamins and minerals. Most gels will provide somewhere between 25-50g of carbohydrate per packet. In this case, the highly concentrated, highly osmotic "gue" needs plenty of water to dilute the contents and facilitate gastric emptying and absorption. For the most part 12 oz of water will help digest these gels. Do not experiment with foods, food supplements, or sports drinks the day of the competition because your performance will drop or, what is worse, might come to a halt.

- *Events lasting longer than 3 hours* – here the main concerns include water, carbohydrates, and electrolytes, especially sodium. The longer sporting events including marathons, Iron Man and Half Iron Man Triathlons, cycling road races fall within this category. Never underestimate longer, non-competitive events such as the 100 to 150-mile tours or 3-4 hour biking, particularly during hot and humid summer days. Water and electrolyte losses, and glycogen depletion will become a nightmare and if not aggressively corrected can lead to very serious and life threatening situations. During these lengthy athletic events, competitive or not, two clinical conditions are seen, not infrequently: Dilutional hyponatremia and "bonking or hitting the wall."

Dilutional hyponatremia – "Water intoxication," better known as hyponatremia, is the result of excessive electrolyte (particularly sodium) losses from sweat with excessive fluid consumption, particularly of hypotonic fluids or water, at a rate that exceeds the rate of sweat loss. When plasma sodium drops to 130mmol/l, symptoms develop. The lower the sodium, the faster it drops and the longer it remains low, the higher the risk of brain swelling (encephalopathy) and lung swelling (pulmonary edema). With plasma levels less than 125 mmol/l, individuals experience headache, vomiting, fatigue, disorientation and confusion, and difficulty breathing due to water leaking into the air spaces (pulmonary edema). Subsequently with sodium plasma levels of less than 110mmol/l, severe cerebral edema will develop leading to seizures, coma, brain stem herniation, respiratory arrest, and death.

Bonking/hitting the wall – The brain's primary source of glucose is blood sugar, which is available from food (carbohydrate) after absorption, and more readily from liver glycogen. Carbohydrate consumption keeps optimal glycogen stores. Low sugar to the brain behaves very similarly to low oxygen to the brain. Quick action is necessary by consuming a carbohydrate containing solution (sports drinks) that is quickly absorbed from the intestine. Symptoms of low sugar include tiredness, irritability, nausea, dizziness, confusion, and fainting along with poor decision making, lack of coordination, motivation, and visual distortion; worse case scenario, seizures and death. The best strategy to prevent this potentially embarrassing situation, that can mess your sporting event, or even more importantly, your health, is to start your training/competition event with full glycogen stores and eat and drink early and frequently. Carbohydrates are the fuel that your brain and muscles need. Consuming fats and protein will not spare your liver and muscle glycogen stores and while you are constantly reminded of protein-rich bars and gels, your main priority are your high-carbohydrate energy sources.

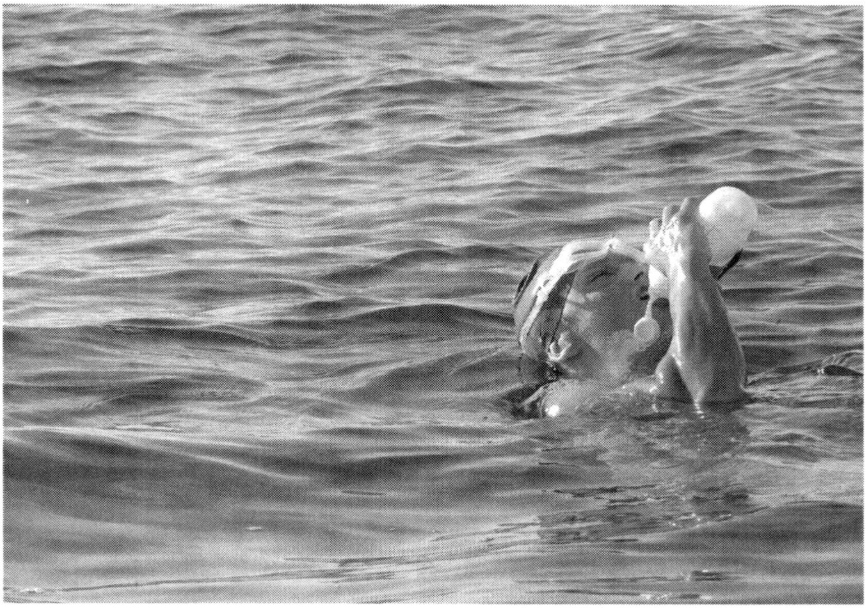

Josh Heynes, male record holder Swim across lake Erie 2006. Nutrition in extreme athletic events is the difference between setting a record or losing a dream. Courtesy of Josh Heynes, MS, ACSM, CEP.

IV. RECOVERY / NUTRITION – HYDRATION

Hydration goal: to replace water and electrolyte losses (i.e., sodium, potassium, calcium, magnesium), correct dehydration and in extreme cases to aggressively intervene with parenteral hydration solutions.

Nutrition goal: to replenish glycogen stores (liver and muscle) in preparation for the next bout of exercise and maintain/replace micro-nutrients required for optimal performance.

How fast you will need to replace fluids and glycogen stores will depend on the length of the recovery intervals between exercise workouts. In a multi-staged sporting event like the Cycling Spring Classics or the Tour de France, where athletes need euhydration and full glycogen tanks the following morning, for one to three consecutive weeks, the hydration and nutritional practices have to be right on schedule and pretty aggressive. In one-day workouts, where recovery periods between sporting events are longer than 72 hours, time allows for a more relaxed approach. The very important "window" of muscle-glycogen re-synthesis, which most experts have estimated take place within the first hour post exercise, is due to increased insulin sensitivity and hence, increased glucose and amino-acid influx across the muscle cell membrane. Carbohydrate consumption during this "window of opportunity," results in higher rates of glycogen storage. High-and-moderate-glycemic index foods are the right choice for the immediate (60 to 90 min) post-exercise nutrition phase particularly to accelerate and optimize muscle glycogen recovery. Liquid forms of carbohydrates provide extra fluids and are easy to digest and better tolerated, especially so, after exhaustive exercise. The recommendations are to consume 1.2g/kg of body weight per hour during the first 4 hours post exercise and a total carbohydrate intake of 8-10g/kg within 24 hours. After the first hour and even more so after 120 minutes, glycogen storage rates can drop significantly. Be aware that protein meals alone will not replenish glycogen stores. In fact, without carbohydrates, muscle recovery is prolonged, taking up to 48-72 hours to recover and, again, assuming that carbohydrate consumption is taking place.

The increased protein synthesis and muscle and tissue repair will take place only when insulin is transporting high glucose loads into the cell along with amino-acids.

Adequate hydration can be achieved by drinking plenty of fluids with electrolytes which, as we have seen, help retain fluids and promptly achieve euhydration. The 2007, ACSM recommendation indicates replacing 1.5 liters of fluid per kg of lost weight. As discussed in Part B, Section IV, under water replacement, this is equivalent to replacing approximately 16 ounces for each pound lost. The fluids consumed should contain approximately 100g of carbohydrate within the first hour post exercise. Hydration and carbohydrate replacement should continue thereafter and, remember, bars and gels cannot substitute for a good meal with plenty of nutritious carbohydrates, proteins, and fluids.

Alcoholic beverages should be taken in moderation, if at all, particularly so with exercise repetitions within less than 12 hours. A glass of wine or a beer can give you a little extra fluid, though there is a diuretic effect with alcoholic beverages if taken in excess. Bottom line, use good judgment and call your priorities.

Health & Fitness

PART D: Body Composition / Energy Balance

I. IDEAL BODY WEIGHT AND BMI (Body Mass Index)

Body weight (mass) and height (stature) are essential measurements readily obtained and utilized for different purposes which include:

a. Determination of human body composition (HBC).
b. Determination of the ideal physique of elite champion athletes.
c. Determination of desirable strength-to-weight ratios for different sport categories.
d. For epidemiologic analysis of quality of life (morbidity) and cause of death (mortality).
e. For prescription of diets and exercise to maintain optimum health.
f. For the accurate administration of therapies and drugs.
g. And many more.

Body weight and mass have been utilized interchangeably and this is also true for height and stature. However, the proper international scientific terms for height (inches), is stature (given in centimeters), and for weight (pounds), is mass (given in kilograms). Based on average ranges of body mass in relation to stature, tables and nomograms have been developed that allow for calculations of "body surface" (m^2) and the "body mass index," the latter which turns out to be a better alternative for calculation of ranges of normalcy in association with body fat composition when compared with an individual measurement like weight or mass.

Body mass index can be calculated using both height (stature) and weight (mass) with the following formulas:

$$BMI = kg \div m^2$$

$$BMI = lb \times 703 \div in^2$$

To convert pounds to kilograms = weight in lb. x 0.45.
To convert inches to centimeters (meters) = height in in. x 0.0254.

The classification of normalcy, underweight, or overweight based on BMI according to the surgeon general definition is seen in table 16.

TABLE 16 SURGEON GENERAL BMI CLASSIFICATION

BMI	CLASS
< 18.5	Underweight
18.5 – 24.9	Normal
25.0 – 29.9	Overweight
30.0 – 39.9	Obese
≥ 40	Morbidly obese

Example 1:
Example of "normal" based on BMI

Male – Mass = 65kg Stature = 1.71m
BMI = 65kg ÷ (1.71m²) = 65 ÷ 2.924 = 22.2

Example 2:
Example of "morbid obesity" based on BMI

Female – Mass = 100kg Stature = 1.52m
BMI = 100kg ÷ (1.52m²) = 100 ÷ 2.3104 = to 43.28

Example 3:
Example of "underweight" based on BMI

Female – Mass = 125 lb Stature = 70 in.
BMI = 125 x 703 ÷ (70 in²) = 87875 ÷ 4900 = 17.93.

Weight and height nomograms as well as the body mass index classification, fail to give accurate determinations of human body composition based on the fat mass and the lean body mass components. The numerator of the BMI classification is affected by lean muscle mass, bone, intracellular and extracellular fluid, in addition to the fat mass component. Two individuals with the same height and weight may have very different fat mass and lean body mass composition. The endurance athlete will have a higher lean muscle mass and the sedentary person will have a lower lean muscle mass, however, a higher fat mass.

Fat plays very important roles. There is fat required for normal physiologic functioning and in fact is sex specific. This type of fat, known as *essential-fat*, is stored in different organ systems including the nervous system, the bone marrow, solid organs like the liver, spleen and kidneys, the heart, skeletal muscle and others.

The other fat accumulates in adipose tissue and plays a very important role as a nutritional reserve. This fat is found surrounding internal organs and mostly appreciated in the subcutaneous tissue. This is known as *storage- fat* with known gender differences. The average normal body fat percentage for physically active young adults, combining both storage-fat and essential-fat is 15% for men and 25% for women. The biggest difference between sexes, however, resides in the essential-fat component which is 3% of body mass for men and 14% of body mass for women. Hence, storage-fat for men is approximately 12% of body weight and 11% for women.

It is important to know that lean body mass still contains the essential fat stores mostly present in the nervous system, bone marrow, and internal organs. Individuals cannot reduce fat below this threshold and still maintain good health.

So what is the ideal body weight? I would like to emphasize that there is an "ideal range" of normalcy and in general we should strive for a body-fat content of no greater than 15 to 20% for men and of no greater than 25-30% for women.

Body composition assessment has been determined utilizing multiple methods which include:

a. Hydrostatic weighing.
b. Measurement of fat folds and body girth.
c. Bioelectrical impedance (BIA).
d. Ultrasound and X-ray (arm fat).
e. Computed tomography (CT) and Magnetic Resonance Imaging (MRI).
f. Dual-Energy X-ray absortiometry (DEXA).
g. BOD-POD (an adaptation of air displacement plethysmography).

The BOD-POD technology is currently available and its accuracy, validity and reproducibility is excellent. The test is easy to administer and takes 3-5 minutes to complete. The individual is seated inside this small air chamber, and based on the known physical relationship between pressure, volume, and temperature (including intrathoracic volumes), measurement of body volume is accurately determined and body fat is calculated. The body composition characteristics of athletes of both sexes in different sport categories have been studied extensively. These studies have incorporated age, height, weight, total body fat, fat free mass, and other measurements. Here is a brief sample of "range of body fat percentages" in different sport categories. Please see table 17.

TABLE 17 RANGE OF BODY FAT PERCENTAGES BASED ON GENDER IN DIFFERENT SPORT CATEGORIES

SPORT	*BODY FAT PERCENTAGES*	
	MALE	**FEMALE**
Long distance running	5-7	15-19
Triathlon	7-8	12-13
All-stroke swimming	5-11	26-27
Cycling	8-9	13-15
Cross country skiing	7-13	15-22

(Modified from Benardot, D. Advanced Sports Nutrition, 2006)

The desirable body mass or weight can be obtained knowing the individuals weight (mass), fat-free mass, and desired fat percentage utilizing the following formula:

Desirable body weight (mass) = fat-free body mass ÷ 1.00 – desired % fat.

1. Weight (mass) in kg or lb.
2. Current percent body fat (i.e., 20% or 0.20).
3. Fat mass in kg or lb = weight x % body fat.
4. Fat-free body mass = weight – fat mass.

5. Using formula as above: desirable body weight (mass).
6. Desirable fat loss = current weight – desirable weight.

Most of these formulas and current technology utilized to determine IBW (ideal body weight) and HBC (human body composition) are very useful for the very reasons stated at the beginning of this section. If we understand our energy balance based on healthy diets and exercise, most problems related with obesity will no longer be a health problem threat.

II. DIET AND EXERCISE (Energy Balance)

Simply stated, the caloric intake should match the caloric expenditure to maintain energy balance, hence body mass (weight). To reduce body mass (weight), either you reduce caloric intake, increase energy expenditure (exercise), or both. It is not my intention to review the scientific literature on obesity, but, both dieting and exercise have been recommended for weight control. One of the reasons why most of the many "ultimate diets" fail to maintain weight loss is the clear miss-match of lifestyle and physical activity (exercise). The same can be said about exercise. Excessive food intake (gluttony) with just modest energy expenditure (i.e., walking) breaks the energy balance equation. Individuals of both genders, who lead physically active lifestyles, or who are involved mostly in endurance exercise programs, tend to maintain their energy balance (body weight). There is accumulating evidence that regular exercise is more effective for long-term weight-control than dieting only. Diets fail over 80% of the time. In general, within a year, one-to-two-thirds of the lost weight is regained and almost all of it, by the end of five years.

The total energy expenditure with exercise is directly related to the effectiveness of the exercise program. There is clear evidence of health-related benefits with exercise, including physical, mental, and social well being, as well as disease prevention. A well structured and purposeful exercise program will not work if there is no consistency and commitment. There has to be power of intention. If we believe we're just molecules that come and go, then be it. However, we have to admit that we live in an elegant and intelligent universe. We come from the "source" and will return to the "source." Without trying to give religious connotations, we should strive to make the best of our human physicality through our human spirituality during this brief journey that we call life on planet earth.

Who are we?

Where do we come from?

Where are we going?

These questions have been with us and will remain with humanity forever. It is my intention that you enjoy the journey. Farewell!

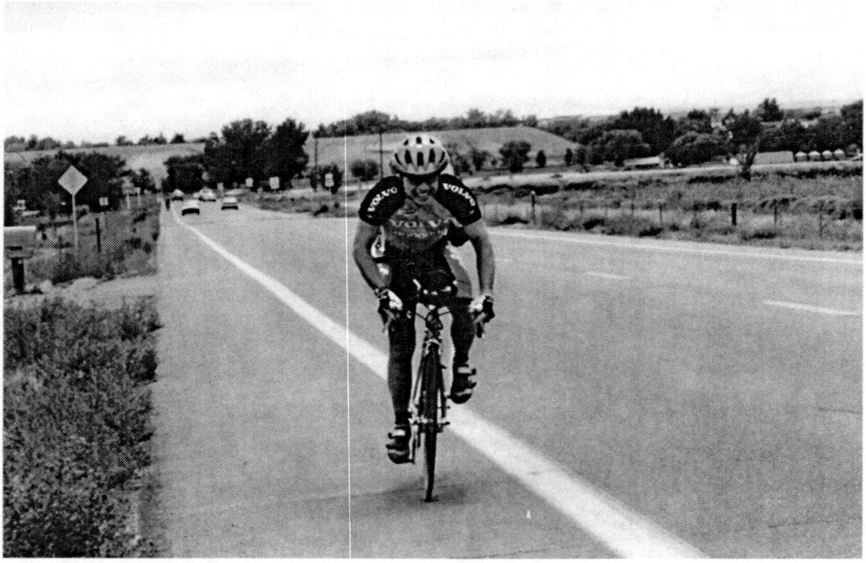

The future belongs to those who believe in the beauty of their dreams -- Eleanor Roosevelt

REFERENCES

- Allen, H., Coggan, A. Training and Racing with a Power Meter. Velo Press, 2005
- American College of Sports Medicine. ACSM's Resource Manual for Guidelines for Exercise Testing and Prescription. Williams and Wilkins, 1998
- Armstrong, L., Carmicheal C. The Lance Armstrong performance program. Rodale, 2000
- Arntz, W., Chasse, B., Vicente, M. What the Bleep do we know!? Health Communication, Inc., 2005
- Australian Sports Commission. AIS Sports supplement program fact sheet: Electrolyte Replacement Supplements. Australian Institute of Sport. Last updated 3/1/07
- Baker, Arnie, M.D. Smart Cycling. New York, NY : Fireside, 1997
- Benardot, D. PhD, RD, FACSM. Advanced Sports Nutrition. Champaign, Il: Human Kinetics, 2006
- Benardot, D. PhD., Thompson, W. PhD. The Coaches' Guide to Sports Nutrition. Coaches Choice. Montery, CA 2007.
- Burke, E.R., PhD. High-Tech Cycling. Champaign, Il : Human Kinetics, 1996
- Burke, E.R., PhD. Serious Cycling. Champaign, Il : Human Kinetics, 2002
- Burke, L., Deakin, V. Clinical Sports Nutrition. McGraw-Hill Australia Co., Inc. 2006
- Capra, F. El Tao de la Fisica (Original title: The Tao of Physics). Editorial Sirio. Málaga, España. 2005
- Capra, F. The Hidden Connections. Doubleday. New York, NY, 2002
- Carmicheal, Chris. Food for Fitness. New York, NY : Penguin Group, 2004
- Carmichael, Chris. The Ultimate Ride. New York, NY: Penguin Group, 2003
- Chopra, D. Life After Death: The Burden of Proof. Harmony Books. New York, NY, 2006

- Chopra, D. The Book of Secrets: Unlocking the Hidden Dimensions of Your Life. Harmony Books, New York, NY, 2004
- Chopra, D. The Spontaneous Fulfillment of Desire: Harnessing the Infinite Power of Coincidence. Harmony Books, New York, NY, 2003
- Dr. Wayne W. Dyer. The Power of Intention: Learning to Co-Create Your World Your Way. Hay House, Inc., 2004
- Edwards, S., Reed, S. Heart Zones Cycling: The Avid Cyclist's Guide to Riding Faster and Farther. Velo Press, 2006
- Gore, CJ. Australian Sports Commission. Physiological Tests for Elite Athletes. Champaign Il: Human Kinetics, 2000
- Greene, B. The Elegant Universe: Superstrings, Hidden Dimensions and the Quest for the Ultimate Theory. Vintage Books, New York, NY, 2003
- Jackobson, Troy. Spinervals Cycling Workout with Coach Troy. Available in Video and DVD. www.coachtroy.com
- Jansen, P. M.D. Lactate Threshold Training. Champaign, Il : Human Kinetics, 2001
- Jeukendrup, A.E., PhD., editor, High Performance Cycling. Champaign, Il : Human Kinetics, 2002
- Jeukendrup, A.E., PhD., Gleeson Michael, PhD. Sport Nutrition: An Introduction to Energy Production and Performance. Champaign,Il: Human Kinetics, 2004.
- Kearns, B. How Lance does it. McGraw-Hill Co., Inc. 2007
- LeMond, G., Gordis, K. Greg Lemond's complete book of Bicycling. New York, NY : The Berkeley Publishing Company, 1990
- Linder, W. Ciclismo en Ruta : Del aficionado al Professional. Barcelona, Spain: Ediciones Martinez Roca, S.A., 1995
- McArdle, W., Katch, F. Katch, V. Exercise Physiology. Energy, Nutrition, and Human Performance. Williams and Wilkins, 1996.
- McTaggart, L. The Field: The Quest for the Secret Force of the Universe. Harper Collins Publishers, Inc., New York, NY, 2002
- Mellion, M.B., M.D., Burke, E.R., PhD. "Bicycling Injuries": Clinics in Sports Medicine. Philadelphia, PA: W.B. Sanders, 1994

- Sawka, M., Burke, L., Eicher, R., et al. American College of Sports Medicine position stand. Exercise and Fluid Replacement. Med. Sci. Sports Exerc.: pg 377-390, 2007
- Scientific American. Special Edition: The Frontiers of Physics. Scientific American Volume 15, No 3, 2005
- Thompson, P.P, M.D. Exercise and Sports Cardiology. McGraw-Hill Co, Inc. 2001
- Tipton, CM., Sawka, M., Tate, C., Terjung, R. ACSM'S: Advanced Exercise Physiology, Lippincott Williams and Wilkins, 2006
- Viru, A., Viru, M. Biochemical Monitoring of Sport Training. Champaign Il: Human Kinetics, 2001
- Willett, W.C., M.D., Eat, Drink and be Healthy: The Harvard Medical School Guide to Healthy Eating. Free Press, A. Division of Simon and Schuster, Inc., New York, NY, 2001

About the Author

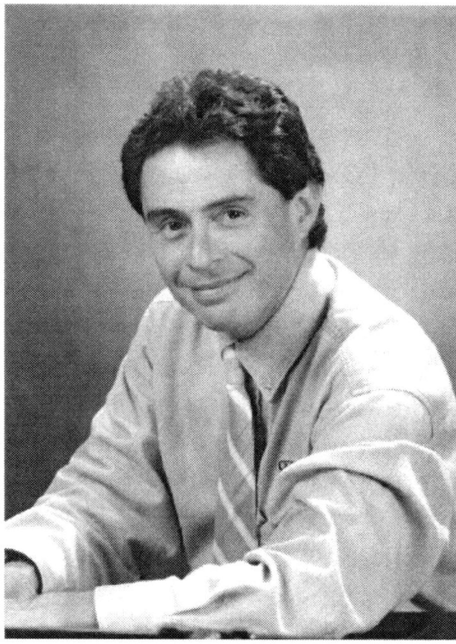

Manuel F. Forero was born in Bogotá, Colombia, October 18, 1956. There, he graduated from Juan N. Corpas, School of Medicine in December 1980. He completed a residency in Family Medicine in Bogotá and relocated to the United States where he completed a residency in Internal Medicine and subsequently a fellowship in Cardiovascular Disease, both at Tulane University affiliated hospitals in New Orleans, Louisiana. Currently he is in private practice and an active invasive and non-invasive cardiologist at Saint Vincent Heart Center in Erie, PA. He is also a certified USA cycling coach.

In one way or another, throughout his life he has been involved in sports. During his early years track and soccer were his main interests. Subsequently he developed a passion for cycling and 16 years later he is still very involved in the sport. He has logged thousands of miles on his legs and hundreds of thousands of hours in the medical field and cardiovascular disease. He has built a solid experience in human cardiopulmonary and exercise physiology and pathophysiology having performed thousands of stress tests using the treadmill and bicycle ergometers with the use of echocardiography, radionuclide imaging, and cardiac catheterization.

He has witnessed and toured during two editions of Le Tour de France (2002 and 2004) and several tours in the United States including, "The Bicycle Tour of Colorado," "Pedal Pennsylvania," and his own "Climb to the Summit" in the Big Island of Hawaii. He has also participated in fund raising events: "Ride for the Roses" in Austin, Texas, for the Lance Armstrong Cancer Foundation and the "MS 150 Bike Tour" in Pittsburgh, PA for multiple sclerosis.

For 27 years he has talked to patients about healthy lifestyle, diet habits, and the benefits of exercise. He believes deeply in the health-related benefits of exercise and good nutrition including physical, mental, and social well being, as well as disease prevention. He insists in the power of intention..... without commitment and consistency no program will work.

"We should strive to make the best of our human physicality through our human spiritually during this brief journey that we call life on planet Earth."

Printed in the United States
107879LV00002B/34/P